PRAISE FOR
Dr. Dean Mitchell's Allergy and Asthma Solution:

"Dr. Mitchell's book is an important new step forward to the best diagnosis and treatment of allergies, and I'm sure it will be a very good basis for any doctor interested in a real update in the field."

—Giorgio Walter Canonica, MD,
Department of Internal Medicine,
University of Genoa (Italy),
World Allergy Organization

Dean Mitchell, MD, is the leading expert in sublingual allergy immunotherapy in the United States. He had been in practice for seven years following the conventional methods of allergy cures when he first learned of sublingual allergy immunotherapy (allergy drops) and has been one of its strongest proponents. He now runs a private practice, Ocean Allergy & Nutrition, in Manhattan. Dr. Mitchell's patients come from all over the United States to receive his treatments. He is a fellow of the American College of Allergy, Asthma, and Immunology and is a member of the Joint Council of Allergy and Immunology. For ten years he was a clinical instructor of medicine at Columbia College of Physicians and Surgeons. He graduated from Brown University in 1982 and received his MD from the Sackler School of Medicine at Tel Aviv University in 1986. He lives in Long Island with his wife and two sons. When he's not busy with his patients, he enjoys playing tennis with his sons.

Dr. Dean Mitchell's
ALLERGY
AND
ASTHMA
SOLUTION

Dr. Dean Mitchell's
ALLERGY
AND
ASTHMA
SOLUTION

THE ULTIMATE PROGRAM FOR REVERSING YOUR SYMPTOMS ONE DROP AT A TIME

DEAN MITCHELL, MD

Marlowe & Company
New York

Dr. Dean Mitchell's Allergy and Asthma Solution:
The Ultimate Program for Reversing Your Symptoms One Drop at a Time

Copyright © 2006 by Dean Mitchell

Published by
Marlowe & Company
An Imprint of Avalon Publishing Group, Incorporated
245 West 17th Street • 11th Floor
New York, NY 10011-5300

AVALON
publishing group incorporated

Library of Congress Cataloging-in-Publication Data

Mitchell, Dean, MD
   Dr. Dean Mitchell's allergy and asthma solution : the ultimate program for reversing your symptoms one drop at a time / Dean Mitchell.
     p. cm.
    1. Allergy—Treatment—Popular works. 2. Asthma—Treatment
—Popular works.   I. Title.
   RC584.M58 2006
   616.97'06—dc22

2006011864

ISBN-10: 1-56924-341-7
ISBN-13: 978-1-56924-341-1

9 8 7 6 5 4 3 2 1

All illustrations except those of chapter 11 © copyright Justin Marler .
Illustrations on pages 160–180 © copyright Kajiah Jacobs.

Book design by Maria E. Torres
Printed in the United States of America

Contents

To my wife, Ricki, an extraordinary mother and doctor. This book is for you and all the other physicians who don white coats each day to help their patients.

Note to My Readers

I feel it is important to inform my readers, as I do all my patients that allergy vaccines in the United States are currently FDA approved for injections, and that giving the vaccine sublingually is considered off-label use. Off-label use means physicians can prescribe any medication for any condition for which it is believed safe and effective based on the supporting medical literature. The allergy vaccines used sublingually are made from the same vaccines used for the injections, the only difference is that the vaccine is taken in drops under the tongue. In general, safety of a medication increases as you go from injections to oral or topical preparations.

Preface

I have been a practicing allergist in New York for the past fifteen years after training at the Robert Cooke Allergy Institute in New York City, an affiliate of Columbia University, College of Physicians and Surgeons. The Cooke Institute is one of the original training programs in the country and has trained allergist who practice all over the country. The training emanated from the work of Dr. Cooke himself, a world-renowned allergist, and involved allergy skin tests with needles and allergy shots; Dr. Cooke's work influenced the practice of allergy for decades up to the present day. I was trained in this same methodology; however, that all changed one fateful day when near tragedy and serendipitous information collided and changed the way I would practice allergy forever.

I'll tell you more about my story later, but first let me share my excitement over this new allergy treatment. This is not just some new medication, promising momentary relief from the symptoms of allergy. The shelves are already brimming with those medications and allergy sufferers are already well acquainted with them—along with their side effects, and the fact that these aids can offer only temporary relief at best. Nor am I referring to the much-dreaded allergy shots, which is the heavy artillery of traditional allergy treatment, reserved for allergy's worst cases. While the shots do help, patient compliance is often tricky, since weekly trips to the doctor (to get a shot!) are no fun.

No, the news I wish to spread with this book is about something altogether different. This is not a "quick fix" medication that merely suppresses the symptoms of allergy to give patients temporary relief—it is a genuine, breakthrough treatment. The difference is that it does not target the symptoms, but rather eradicates the underlying condition that gives rise to allergic symptoms in the first place. By addressing the underlying condition, you can actually stop the symptoms *before* they occur. It is the difference between taking something to lessen the symptoms of a terrible cold, and taking something that will cure your cold. And here's the best part, not only does a treatment for allergy exist, but it is simple, painless, and can be done in your own home—and for a large majority of people it can stop the suffering.

Too good to be true? No. With so many headlines sending consumers so many mixed health messages these days, and with so much hype being generated to sell so many products—both over-the-counter and by prescription—promising to treat so many maladies, a healthy skepticism is certainly warranted. That's why I want you to know that I am a traditionally trained medical doctor who believes that any time the hype around a product is not backed by rigorous, sound medical science, then buyer beware.

In the pages that follow I will tell you in greater detail about how I came to learn about this well-kept secret, but let me assure you that this treatment is real, and backed by thorough, rigorous science. I became so confident in the scientific evidence supporting this treatment that I began using it with my patients—and the results are nothing short of stunning. So, in addition to the science, I've also witnessed the clinical proof first hand, and I'll share that with you as well.

Seeing the spectacular results with my own patients is what led to the writing of this book. Seeing truly is believing. Yet as an individual clinician I can treat only so many patients, and as happy as I am to be helping my own patients with this new treatment, I began to feel a responsibility as well to the public at large. Since the treatment remains such a secret, unheard of by most allergy sufferers and allergists alike, I didn't feel I could sit by as millions of people suffer unnecessarily.

I've written this book to be used in several ways: However, as with any patient-doctor office visit, the greatest benefit occurs when both parties work together. In this book I will teach you the ideas and language to help you better understand how your allergies and asthma develop, and will offer specific ways for you to be proactive in taking control of your allergies and asthma. For example, I will discuss an Asthma Action Plan that teaches you how to assess and regulate your asthma and will share the Better Breathing Program— a chapter for readers who want to optimize their health with special breathing exercises.

So I write this book as both your greatest advocate and as a medical reporter of sorts, in order to spread the word about what I consider to be the single most important breakthrough in the treatment of allergy—a truly effective cure: sublingual allergy immunotherapy, or allergy drops.

Introduction

If you're reading this book, you are likely one of 31 million people in the United States who suffer from allergies, or one of 16 million asthma sufferers. Or perhaps you have a loved one who you see struggling on a beautiful spring or fall day because of the high pollen counts, or who can't visit the homes of friends or relatives because they sneeze or wheeze around the family pets. If you or someone close to you are tired of the sneezing, the sniffling, the watery eyes or the wheezing—and of the constraints imposed on you by your allergy—then you've found the right book.

People ask me how I can be writing a book while tending to a busy clinical practice. I have no choice: I am so gratified by the results I see from this revolutionary treatment to reverse allergies and asthma, that I truly feel a bit like a missionary on a crusade, eager to get out the good news, not only to my own patients, but to every adult and child who is suffering from allergy or asthma.

The field of allergy and asthma has evolved a great deal over the last twenty-five years, although unfortunately many of the old practices are still in fashion—even though the number of asthma cases in the United States has quadrupled. While advances in medicine have thrust us forward and enabled us to treat so many other diseases and health conditions, and although we are able to successfully *treat* the growing numbers of asthma cases emerging, the problem is that we are seeing more and more new asthma sufferers.

I decided to write this book to bring this important message directly to the millions of people who suffer from allergy and asthma. *Dr. Dean Mitchell's Allergy and Asthma Solution* is not only a guide to help you understand *why* you have allergies and/or asthma, but it also introduces a new, breakthrough therapy, backed by solid science, that has been shown conclusively to *reverse* allergies and asthma! That's right, this treatment does not merely target the symptoms of allergy, but it acts upon the mechanism that gives rise to allergy in the first place. For most allergy and asthma sufferers, it can actually help turn your condition around, permanently. This revolutionary new therapy is called *sublingual allergy immunotherapy*, or *allergy drops* in plain English, and it is a breakthrough treatment that has already been available in Europe for the past twenty-five years. Now it has finally emerged in American medicine with the same promise of safety and effectiveness. In a certain sense, it is truly the best of all possible worlds, a new discovery that isn't *new* at all and thus has the advantage of boasting twenty-five years of good results in the field.

So if this treatment is really so great, you are probably wondering, *then why did it take so long to bring it to the United States?* That's a long story, and I'll share my own small role in this. For me, the story begins when I, by chance, learned about allergy drops from a veteran allergist in the Midwest. Dr. David Morris defied the conventional allergists for two decades, but he faced a sea of opposition as he tried to change the mindset and the clinical practice of allergy treatment in the United States. He might not have succeeded in getting the word out, but he did succeed in helping a remarkable number of lucky allergy patients who had the good fortune to come to him for care.

This book is written as a result of my initial discovery of Dr. Morris, my experiences watching him work, and my clinical experience over the past decade treating patients with allergies and asthma and using the allergy drops to help improve their lives. Historically, the field of allergy has been viewed with deep skepticism by the public and also by physicians in other subspecialties. Sometimes with good cause, many people thought that allergy treatment was quackery. For example, a standard treatment in the 1950s and '60s was for the patient to vacuum the house dust in his home and bring it to the allergist, who would then make up a "serum" (the old term for allergy vaccine) and give the patient weekly injections of dirt from his own home in order to desensitize him to his household dust. Patients weren't thrilled about this, and doctors in other specialties thought the technique was ludicrous. However, to everyone's surprise, many patients reported benefit from this treatment. The naysayers, of course, said it was simply the placebo effect; but years later, researchers at several institutions, including Johns Hopkins, showed that inside the house dust were dust mites, which stimulated immune protection to the dust.

With this advancement, the field of allergy began to gain respectability and the demand for allergy shots grew dramatically, as they were the only available source of relief besides antihistamines. Allergy shots, however, proved to be a less than perfect solution. Patients weren't thrilled about getting injections every week, year after year. The shots can be painful. Some patients' arms would swell up for days after the injection. They sometimes wondered if the treatment was worth it, and sometimes decided that living with their allergic symptoms was preferable. Aside from the inconvenience of weekly visits to the doctor's office, there was no end of treatment in sight. Normally patients are accustomed to following a prescribed course of treatment for an ailment, like a course of antibiotics to treat an infection, let's say, where one can expect at the end of ten days to be finished with medication and free of infection. Yet in the case of allergies, many patients were told they would need these injections for the rest of their lives. When I was a resident and was accepted into my hospital's allergy fellowship, an attending doctor who was trying to entice me away from allergy and to instead choose to go into his own specialty of gastroenterology said, "Allergy—isn't that the field of medicine where you don't kill anybody, but you don't ever *cure* anybody, either?"

Today nothing could be further from the truth. You can be allergy free! You will learn in the pages that follow how sublingual allergy immunotherapy, "allergy drops," are safer than allergy shots, more convenient, and offer long-term protection for both allergies and asthma. These groundbreaking allergy drops are in the literal sense a solution for allergy sufferers: they are the natural allergens in a glycerin base. They work because they are a solution that stimulates the immune system to tolerate and protect against the environment's airborne allergens without the side effects of drugs. As Dr. Steve Salvatore from New York City's Fox News 5 reported, "It's a treatment that's easy to swallow."

But you won't simply learn more about your own condition in these pages; you'll also see how dozens of people, just like you, have enjoyed real-life success stories. I want you to discover for yourself just how dramatically your life can be improved, and to do so I will share with you some of the stories of my own patients.

I have also included a chapter on conditions that can masquerade or mimic allergies or asthma. You might be tempted to skip this chapter because you think you already *know* that you have allergies or asthma. Or you may think, "Because I've already been tested and the doctor says it's my allergies, there's no doubt." Please don't skip this section. Even an experienced physician can sometimes be fooled and may occasionally diagnose allergy when it is actually something else. The longer I am in practice, the more I try to remember the medical saying, "When you hear the sounds of hoofbeats, you don't tend to think of zebras." The zebras, not the horses, are the unusual diagnosis.

Finally, I have created a simple, easy-to-follow program that will show you how to enjoy better breathing. The Better Breathing Program evolved from my training at some of the best centers in the country for holistic medicine. It is a multiple-step protocol based on the science of mind-body medicine and the emerging field of psychoneuroimmunology. In the program, you will learn how to determine your stress-level "score" and how to reduce that score. The steps you'll follow fall under two categories: the first set incorporates breathing exercises that have been in Eastern medicines for centuries to relieve the stress and tension in your body and reduce difficulty breathing through your nose, sinuses, and chest. The second part of the program integrates stretching exercises that are similar to basic yoga postures that will open up the neck, chest, pelvis, and spine—ultimately making breathing easier.

It is important to remember that there are many components of this program that may work for you, but others that may not. Learn as much as you can so you can work in partnership with your physician to get optimal results.

CHAPTER

1

What Are Allergies?

I'm excited about sharing this new breakthrough cure for allergies, because I know how devastating allergies can be and how they affect the quality of everyday living. But before you can fully appreciate how revolutionary this treatment really is, you'll want to understand a bit about what happens when your body has an allergic reaction. Understanding why you sneeze, wheeze, or suffer from watery eyes when exposed to certain allergens will help you to better comprehend why and how allergy drops not only stop the symptoms, but the underlying condition that causes those symptoms as well.

The Basics of Allergies

An allergic reaction is what happens when your body's immune system *overreacts* to a benign substance, such as tree pollen or pet dander. In other words, your body responds by going into attack mode against an agent that it erroneously perceives as threatening. When the body sounds this alarm, the immune system goes into self-protection mode—launching a vigorous and violent counterattack against potentially harmful intruders, such as pollen grains, mold spores, dust mites, animal dander, foods, or certain drugs. That overreaction takes its toll on the body, and can be likened to getting out the heavy artillery when you're battling a common housefly.

The single most important fact when learning about allergies is something that Dr. Vincent Beltrani of Columbia University impressed upon me when I was beginning my training to become an allergist: "You're never allergic to something the *first* time you get exposed to it." As a physician who treats allergy patients, I find myself having to repeat this mantra over and over again, not only to my patients, but also to fellow doctors to whom I lecture. This reality is sometimes hard to grasp and is counterintuitive; we tend to think it is white or black—someone is either allergic or not. That's why almost every time you encounter a person with a food allergy, they are perplexed and invariably say something like: "How can I possibly be allergic to shrimp? I've eaten it a thousand times!" Well, that's my point, it was the thousand and first time that did the trick and triggered the trip wire of an allergic reaction.

So what determines that "tipping point"? Over time, and by repeated exposure, the body's immune system can become "sensitized" so that the body will no longer tolerate a certain agent, even though it was fine when it was exposed to that agent before. This can be a frustrating and frightening concept for patients who wonder how this can happen so suddenly.

It's simple, really. The allergen, in this case a food, is introduced to the body's immune system, which now sees the food as a harmful invader, and reacts. The reaction comes out of nowhere, and as surprising and strange as it seems, people do become allergic to precisely those foods that they regularly consume. In the United States, wheat and milk are the most common food allergies. In Japan, it's rice.

The same holds true of inhalant allergies as well. Many of my hay fever patients ask me, "How come I developed this allergy in my thirties?" Again, I explain to them that allergies result over time, and after repeated exposure. The common belief that only children develop allergies, or that most people grow out of their allergies in adulthood, is simply not true.

The Allergic Profile

Although children are by no means the only ones to develop allergies, by observing the development of allergy in children we have gained an important window from which to closely observe the process. We know that children who are genetically predisposed to develop allergic diseases will generally develop symptoms and signs of disease in a predictable sequence throughout childhood. This staged and expected trajectory has been called the *allergic march.*[1]

At intervals, an allergic child will first develop eczema in infancy. This skin condition presents as an itchy, red rash that typically involves the cheeks, neck, chest, and outside surfaces of the arms, legs, and elbows. These infants and young children (under three years old) may also develop gastrointestinal symptoms like colic, diarrhea, and abdominal pain or suffer from chronic ear infections. As the allergic child matures, the skin and gastrointestinal symptoms may subside and give way to respiratory symptoms with the development of nasal congestion and asthma.

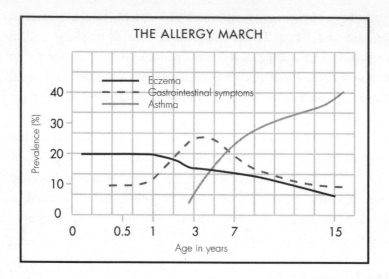

Later on, as we grow toward and through adulthood, allergies cease to follow a straight line, and as a result they are not always easy to spot, so we don't always know that we are allergic, even if the symptoms are in plain view. For example, since allergies present in a different ways, allergic patients may already have seen one or more specialists before they are sent to an allergist. The patients follow the symptoms, which often take them down other paths: they go where it hurts them, not realizing that the actual condition may underlie their symptoms.

The funny thing about allergies is that you don't know when or where they may hit you. Another doctor I trained with once said, "The allergist is the one doctor without an organ to call his own." He meant that a dermatologist is the specialist for the skin; the pulmonologist is the lung doctor; the otolaryngologist is an ear, nose, and throat (ENT) doctor; the ophthalmologist treats the eyes. What's left for the allergist? Well, in truth, the allergist needs to be a specialist in *all* of these areas and must treat the whole patient in order to be effective. Allergists must be generalists, because allergies affect all of these organs, and usually the complaint can be addressed once the underlying allergic cause is identified.

So when someone says, "I have allergies!" he or she can mean a lot of different things, as described in the sidebar titled Where Does It Hurt? But what's more troubling is when a person has one of the allergic conditions and doesn't realize it's due to an allergy. If you're one of those people who seem to have a cold for an entire season, and all of those cold medications aren't working, you just might be treating the wrong malady.

Where Does It Hurt?

The following conditions (including some you may not expect) are commonly caused by allergies:

- *Rhinitis*: This is an inflammation of the nose that causes chronic nasal congestion, sneezing, and runny nose. If it occurs in the fall, we call it hay fever; if it occurs in the spring we call it rose fever. If it lasts all year long, the patients call it "the cold that never goes away."
- *Sinus Problems*: Another part of the nose that is affected by allergies is the sinuses. The sinuses are small air spaces in the skull. They can become inflamed by stagnant airflow or drainage. This can be due to an anatomical problem or an underlying allergic inflammation, which can block the sinuses.
- *Asthma*: Asthma is a very common condition in which a patient may have difficulty breathing, tightness in the chest, or wheezing. The patient can also present with a chronic "tight" cough that hasn't responded to antibiotics. It has been clearly shown that allergics play a large role in triggering asthma.
- *Eczema and Hives*: These are two common skin conditions that are frequently exacerbated by allergies. Eczema has been shown to flare up in patients after they have eaten certain foods or have

continues

been exposed to environmental allergens. Hives can be caused
by foods such as fish, nuts, or berries. Medications are also well
known to cause hives—even if the patient has used them before
without a problem.

• *Blepharitis and Conjunctivitis*: Commonly associated with swelling of
the eyelids and itchy, watery eyes. These symptoms are frequently
due to airborne particles like pollens, molds, and animal dander.

Allergy Triggers

Listed below are the four main types of allergies and how they affect
your body's immune system.

Airborne Allergies

An airborne allergic response begins after a particle in the air, such
as dust, pollen, mold, or animal dander, is inhaled through the nose,
where it can then lodge or travel farther down the respiratory tract
into the lungs. At some point in the journey, the allergen,
depending on its size, binds to your nasal or lung tissue and an
immune response is triggered.

Outdoor Allergens

• *Pollens* are outdoor allergens and are the best known
because they affect so many people every spring and
fall. The spring pollens mainly include the different
trees and grasses that pollinate beginning in March
and lasting until June. The classic highest pollen days
for spring pollens in the northeastern United States
are between Mother's Day and Memorial Day. The
major fall pollen, ragweed, actually begins to rise in
mid-August, usually peaks around Labor Day
weekend, and finally subsides by mid-October.

Indoor Allergens

- *Dust mites* are by far the most frequent trigger of indoor allergies. These microscopic organisms are found in *everyone's* bedding—pillows, blankets, and mattresses—and carpeting and can cause a lot of problems, including asthma and eczema. Note: you can be the most expert housekeeper, but no matter how clean a house you keep, all bedding has dust mites.

- *Household pets* are another major source of indoor allergies. Yes, cats and dogs are a major cause of allergies. While we take that for granted today, for many years doctors and patients were in disbelief that a cat could cause someone to have asthma. But today the cat allergen has been identified as *Fel d 1*.

- *Cockroaches* are generally despised, but now you have even more reason to loathe them: the cockroach allergen. Study after study has shown that the cockroach allergen is a major cause of inner-city asthma. Cockroaches don't discriminate based on your bank account, but rather on the conditions where you work or live. If you live in a turn-of-the-century home or apartment, you need to check to make sure that cockroaches don't lurk in your walls or heating systems. Cockroaches also love to creep around around the kitchen sink, so don't leave dishes lying around with food particles on them or let the faucets drip.

Indoor/Outdoor Allergens

- *Molds* are a significant cause of both indoor and outdoor allergens. You've probably seen newspaper headlines about how toxic mold made people sick and destroyed homes after the Hurricane Katrina disaster. But more commonly, mold grows in homes that have been affected by excess moisture, and its presence can lead to respiratory allergies: sinus inflammation and asthma. Mold is also an outdoor allergen and is becoming a growing problem that is frequently overlooked when allergic reactions occur. The peak time for mold allergies is in the heat of the summer when it's humid and mold spores release into the air—much like when leaves fall from the trees and decompose in the fall.

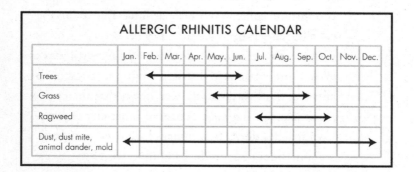

Food Allergies

Any food can trigger an allergic response. In the United States the most common allergy-inducing foods are milk, wheat, eggs, soy, fish, and nuts. Any of these foods can bring on a variety of symptoms, from a stomachache to a rash or even difficulty in breathing—and, in extreme cases, death.

Unlike other allergies, there is no treatment for food allergies—only strict avoidance of the allergen. Food allergies can also be confused with food intolerances, such as lactose intolerance, but are not the same. A person with intolerance for milk can consume it and may have uncomfortable side effects, such as bloating or a stomachache, but the milk will not cause an immune response. Many patients come to my office wondering why they've suddenly developed a reaction to a food they've eaten all their lives. To explain developed food allergies, I'll share my experience with the "pizza man." A patient came to my office who was the spitting image of the man on the cover of a pizza box: jet black hair and a handlebar mustache. However, this was a very sad-looking pizza man. He was concerned because every time he ate pizza or pasta he developed a rash and had difficulty breathing. He couldn't understand it: since he was seventeen years old, he had been making and eating pizza. What was going on?

I conducted the specific food tests, and the results explained everything. The pizza man was allergic to the wheat from which he made his pizza crusts! This "sudden" allergy was actually the result of a predisposition to a wheat allergy, combined with all those years of exposure touching and breathing in wheat flour, and of course from eating his delicious pizzas.

Your Immune System's Role in Allergies

As discussed earlier, an allergic reaction is your body's way of putting up a quick barrier against a perceived threat. So now you know that anything from eating a slice of pizza to putting your head down on your favorite pillow might trigger an allergic reaction, but what happens *exactly* when an allergic response occurs? To better understand the allergic response, as I suggested at the start of this chapter, it helps to learn a few simple basics about the immune system— your body's first line of defense.

The immune system is our primary defense against hostile attack from a host of potential enemies, like bacteria, viruses, and even cancer. The immune system is also the mechanism *responsible for* our response to allergens. But while the mechanism is the same, why is it that our bodies mount a defensive attack against something as benign as a blade of grass, some pet dander, or pollen? Seemingly, these benign agents are not posing the sort of threat that viruses and bacteria do, so why the strong reaction?

The truth is we don't know for sure *why* this reaction occurs, but we do know a great deal about *how* it occurs. So let's take a closer look at what happens on the cellular level.

The Pieces of the Puzzle: The Allergic Cells of the Immune System

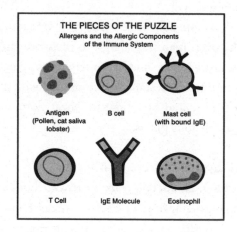

The human immune system is made up of white blood cells produced from our bone marrow. The white cells are divided into different components: *neutrophils, lymphocytes, monocytes, eosinophils, basophils,* and natural killer cells. The lymphocytes are divided into two main groups: *T-cells* (*T* standing for cells that are derived from the bone marrow but that mature in the thymus gland around the neck) and *B-cells* (produced and matured in the bone marrow).

T-cells are the main orchestra of the immune system. They "direct" traffic in how our immune system should defend against a foreign substance. B-cells are directed by the T-cells to produce antibodies, which bind to their foreign substances and designate them for destruction by the natural killer cells of the immune system. Eosinophils and basophils, colorful cells when looked at under the microscope, are not important in the daily life of the immune system—unless you have allergies. Some people have a mistaken image of the immune system as a group of Pac-Man-like cells that indiscriminately flow through our bloodstream, gobbling up any organisms that float by and are identified as "not us." In fact, the human immune system is strategically astute, as it has evolved over thousands of years to become a highly sophisticated defense operation.

I prefer to think of the immune system not along the lines of Pac-Man, but as grand master chess wizard. As in chess, our immune system is comprised of different players, each with their specific moves and functions. Any person who has played chess knows that pawns, rooks, knights, bishops, kings, and queens each have different roles and values in the game. A pawn is sent out to do a small job, while the more powerful pieces, located behind the row of pawns, await more complicated missions. Similarly, our immune system is set up to have an appropriately *measured* response.

When confronted by an opponent, the immune system first engages its pawns to dispense of minor threats to our health and saves the heavy artillery—its rooks, bishops, knights, and so forth—

for a more formidable foe. One of the most fascinating aspects of the human immune system is that it gets wiser with each engagement. Each time that it attacks an intruder (bacteria, virus, and so forth) it downloads a profile of relevant information about the interloper—and can hold on to that information for decades. Should any reexposure from that same trespasser occur, it will be dealt with swiftly and efficiently.

For decades, patients who had allergies were said to have reaginic *antibodies* in their blood—meaning researchers could transfer their blood to another patient and elicit an allergy reaction by a skin test. But no one knew what this reaginic antibody was. We now understand that this mysterious antibody in allergic people is *IgE (Immunoglobulin E)*. IgE was discovered by Drs. Teruko and Kimishige Ishizaka at a Denver hospital in the late 1960s. The revelation by this husband-and-wife team was nothing short of groundbreaking: this key component, found in the blood, sets off the cascade of reactions that leads to an allergic reaction when bound to an allergen.[2]

Shaped like a capital Y, this "allergy antibody" was also later found to be present in the nose, lung, and even skin, which explained why allergy skin tests worked in identifying allergies. (These skin tests were reliable, but how they worked had remained a mystery for almost a hundred years.) The ability to quantify a patient's IgE in a lab test gives doctors a good idea of how allergic the patient is. However, technology in blood testing has become so sophisticated that a lab test can now identify how strong a child's or adult's allergies are to specific allergens, such as cat, dog, or other airborne particles. This, we will see, is important in predicting who will develop significant allergies and asthma.

What Is Sensitization?

Before an allergic reaction can occur, your body must be sensitized to an allergen. Remember, you're never allergic the first time you eat a certain food or take a medication, because you haven't become sensitized yet. For allergen sensitization the following four steps must occur:

1. Tiny particles (the allergen), like dust, mold, or animal dander float in the air and are inhaled; or in the case of a food or drug, are eaten and digested.
2. The immune system reacts by producing specific "allergy antibodies" called *specific IgE* (meaning specific to each allergen dog or cat).
3. The IgE antibodies bind to receptors on the surface of the mast cells (boat cells that carry the IgE in the blood or anchor them in the lining of the skin or mucus membranes).
4. Now your body is sensitized. The next time you're exposed to the allergen, your body can unleash the full allergic response.

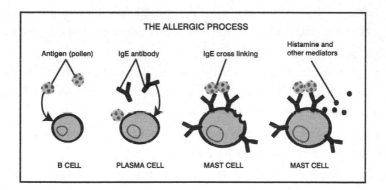

THE ALLERGIC PROCESS

Antigen (pollen)   IgE antibody   IgE cross linking   Histamine and other mediators

B CELL   PLASMA CELL   MAST CELL   MAST CELL

IgE and Childhood Asthma

It is now believed that testing IgE in young children can be a good predictor of which children will develop asthma later on in life. The groundbreaking work of Dr. Fernando Martinez and his team at the University of Arizona at Tucson have shown that the total IgE can be measured both in placental blood and in children at nine months of age. He showed that the total IgE measured at nine months of age was a good predictor as to which children would go on to develop asthma.[3]

A new study from England and Sweden went a step further. Researchers wanted to see if by measuring IgE they could predict which children under five years of age who had an episode of wheezing would be persistent "wheezers" at age five. The researchers measured the children's specific IgE levels to dust mites and to cat and dog allergens. They found that for children with higher levels of these three allergens, specific IgE was a reliable predicator of which children would still be wheezing at five years of age. They also found that higher specific IgE levels to dust mite, cat, and dog allergens were associated with lower levels of lung function in these children. This finding applied only to these specific airborne allergens: dust mite, cat, and dog—it wasn't affected by food-specific IgE, such as peanut allergen.[4]

My best advice to you is to find out your child's specific IgE levels if he or she has had an episode of wheezing. Many children can have an episode of wheezing from a respiratory infection. However, if wheezing is recurrent, it would be prudent to do the simple test to determine if they are likely to develop asthma.

The following sections about two other players in the immune process may also be helpful to you, and I've tried to simplify the ideas as much as possible. The important thing to take away from the discussion of these two cells is that they can provide valuable information to your doctor about how severe your allergies and asthma are, how they may develop, and what can be done to treat them.

Eosinophil

While our understanding of IgE has revolutionized the field of allergies, there's another major player on the scene—the eosinophil cell—whose importance has only recently come to be known. There is a great irony in the fact that these cells are now taking a central role in allergy diagnosis and treatment, since for many years they were regarded as the "forgotten cells" by doctors and researchers. (As I mentioned, these cells are present in everyone, but usually in such a small number as to be insignificant in the everyday functioning of the immune system.)

The eosinophil cell is a component of the immune system's white blood cells. When scientists use their basic stains to look at cells under the microscope, this cell appears with bright red dots filled throughout its contents.[5] In medical school we were taught that if a patient had an elevated total eosinophil count, it signified "worms, wheezes, or weird diseases." The "worms" part meant that a high eosinophil count could represent a parasitic infection. Fortunately, parasitic infections are uncommon today in the Western world. However, they are still prevalent in Third World countries. This helps us understand how the eosinophil might have been an important cell in fighting infections before good hygiene and before antibiotics. However, through the evolution of our immune systems and the discovery of powerful medications, this cell's function began to be perceived as obsolete.

Yet we now know that eosinophils play an important role in allergic conditions. The second word from the above adage, "wheezes," notes the importance of the eosinophil in the clinical finding of a wheezing patient, which usually means someone with asthma. It hasn't been until the last decade that doctors and researchers began to understand how important and powerful a cell the eosinophil is in orchestrating allergic conditions such as asthma and allergic rhinitis and sinusitis. This cell not only circulates in the bloodstream, but it can also infiltrate tissue in the nose and lungs to cause inflammation.[6]

Once researchers understood that the powerful allergy medications called *corticosteroids* blocked the action and migration of eosinophils, they began to incorporate them successfully in topical preparations of nose sprays and inhalers to give rhinitis and asthma sufferers relief. We will further discuss the role of eosinophils on asthma and sinusitis in later chapters.

T-Cells

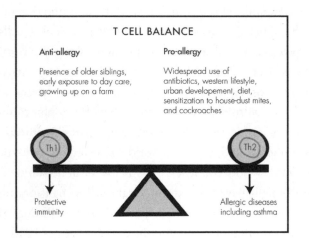

Finally, one of the biggest breakthroughs in understanding allergies has been the discovery of the different types of T-cells. The word *T-cells* has almost become common lingo with the AIDS epidemic. T-cells are one of the two main types of cells that make up the white blood count in our bodies and fight infections (the other type is B-cells, which produce antibodies).

The T-cells are critical in orchestrating the body's immune defense; that's why when the T helper cells are destroyed, it wreaks havoc and the patient develops life-threatening infections. Researchers have discovered two main classes of T-cells, which they call *T helper 1* cells and *T helper 2* cells. It has been found that T helper 1 cells help us fight infections. T helper 2 cells cause the body to trigger an allergic response.[7]

Interestingly, researchers have determined that when we are born, the T-cells that predominate in our bodies are the T helper 2 cells—meaning those that cause allergic responses. However, in most infants and children, the T helper 1 cells develop and dominate in response to all the infections children are exposed to. We will see in the next chapter why this explains the prevalence of allergies and how we can shift the balance of the T helper cells to cure allergies.

What Goes Wrong?

Why, then, does the body's sophisticated defense system go haywire when exposed to a mere allergen—a substance that is harmless and poses no actual threat? One theory posits that just as our primitive physical anatomy was designed to help early humans be efficient hunters and gatherers and not to do instant messaging on the computer, researchers speculate that our immune system was designed to fight off what was the most prevalent and worrisome threat at the time: parasites. Parasitic infections, once rampant, are no longer a threat in developed countries with good hygiene, yet they remain a significant threat today in Africa and other underdeveloped countries.

Notably, the immune response to parasitic infection mirrors the allergy response: in both instances we can expect to see an increased production of eosinophil cells and also a certain antibody—Immunoglobulin E. Eosinophils are a component of our blood's white blood cells and are activated in allergic reactions and parasitic infections to defend the body against the "foreign" intruders. Some people believe this shows the Darwinian theory of "survival of the fittest" in action. If your ancestors had an immune system that could efficiently fight off parasitic infections without the aid of antibiotics (which didn't come into existence for many centuries), you and your progeny were at an advantage in the survival sweepstakes. Yet in the twenty-first-century United States and other developed nations, where parasitic infections are now exceedingly rare, your immune system jumps into attack mode in response to a neighbor mowing his lawn or your friend's pet cat climbing up on your lap. And as a result, you may experience the sneezes and wheezes that typify allergy and asthma.

The following mystery to scientists today is why are allergies and asthma so prevalent compared to earlier times. The next chapter gives us some interesting theories.

CHAPTER

2

Why Are Allergies
So Prevalent Today?

My patients frequently ask me, "Are allergies in general becoming more common?" The answer is that indeed they are. Because of this, many of my patients who had never experienced allergies in childhood are perplexed about why they are suffering now as adults.

There is credible scientific evidence to support my assertion that there is a higher incidence of allergy occurring today than ever before. A recent report showed that 54 percent of people between five and fifty-nine years of age had a positive test to at least one allergen.[1] Further, figures from the National Center for Health Statistics indicate that the number of asthma cases in the United States jumped 74 percent from 1980 to 1996![2] These findings correspond with studies from other countries, such as Japan and the United Kingdom.

Global Warming Is Affecting Allergies

The blistering heat wave of summer 2005 was unprecedented in intensity, duration, and geographic reach. More than two hundred U.S. cities registered record-high temperatures that reflected massive ongoing changes in our climate.[3] Since 2001 the pace of atmospheric warming and accumulation of carbon dioxide is quickening. How do such changes affect allergies? Recent research has shown that ragweed grown in conditions with twice the level of carbon dioxide in the air results in 60 percent more pollen.[4] Also, elevated carbon dioxide levels promote the growth of spore production; and with diesel particles from automobiles, these fungi spores can land in the respiratory system and cause an allergic reaction.[5]

With warmer temperatures and more humidity, conditions are perfect for mold growth in soil and on foliage. In recent years, mold spores have taken center stage in terms of what I'm seeing for the first time in my fifteen years of allergy practice.

Molds

What is mold? It is a fungus that lives on dead, decaying material and thrives in warm, damp, moist environments. You've probably seen mold on old bread (that's how penicillin was discovered) or on old rotten fruit (it can appear white, mixed with green and black). You may have seen it on your shower wall in the bathroom or smelled it in your basement (that mildew smell). However, the main sources of outdoor mold are the brown patches of dead grass you see during the scorching days of summer or the piles of golden-brown leaves that fall from your trees in autumn.

The mold grows on these dying organisms and then becomes airborne, which is when it becomes a problem for your respiratory system. The mold spore season typically begins quietly in the spring, reaches a crescendo in the summer, and plateaus through the fall until the first frost. The cold and snow puts the mold into hibernation, and then the cycle begins again the following spring.

Scarecrow Asthma

When Carrie first came to see me, she was a bright and energetic thirty-one-year-old married woman with a three-year-old son. She had a demanding job in advertising that required air travel to other cities at least once a month. When she came to see me, she had a past history of mild, intermittent asthma that responded to an Albuterol inhaler—a medicine that is used to open up the lungs in a patient with chest congestion due to asthma. Carrie's problem now was that her asthma was becoming more persistent, and she noticed that especially in the fall months she would have "wheezing" for a full month.

Carrie made an interesting observation as we discussed her case. Whenever she raked the leaves on her lawn, she developed immediate shortness of breath and needed her inhaler. During our conversation she also recalled another strange event: in October, a few weeks before Halloween, she went to a nursery to pick out a scarecrow to decorate the front yard of her home. After purchasing the scarecrow she put him in the backseat of her car. It was a cold fall day, so all of the car windows were up. Within fifteen minutes of leaving the nursery, Carrie began to experience chest tightness and shortness of breath. She panicked and rolled down the driver's side window, gasping for air. She pulled over to the side of the road and used her asthma inhaler. This gave her enough relief to enable her to drive home. When she got home she checked her *peak flow* (a measurement of air flow in the lungs) and found it was 200. This was 100 points lower than her normal value. She used her inhaler, and within a few hours her breathing had improved.

As she told me this story and filled in other details, I listened carefully and told her my diagnosis: scarecrow asthma. I had never heard of such a case before, but I knew from seeing scarecrows that they are stuffed with hay, and hay is a breeding ground for mold spores. I told Carrie to get rid of the scarecrow (advising her to have someone else tote him away!), but to bring me some clipping from the hay. I sent the material to a lab to be analyzed. Sure enough, the hay had some common molds to which Carrie was highly allergic.

From now on, of course, Carrie could steer clear of scarecrows. But what about every summer and fall when the mold spore counts are high? How would she cope? We had tried allergy injection therapy with her in the past, but she was too sensitive and developed wheezing from the injections and stopped taking them. Then I told her about the new sublingual allergy drops that I've been using in my practice with great success and suggested that she might want to try them for the mold allergy.

Carrie was very interested, since she dreaded the other options. I started her on a low dose of the mold allergy vaccine, and she tolerated it very well without any side effects. Over the course of the year, we reached a maintenance dose, which helped her to develop a tolerance level to the mold. When the next mold spore season began, she had some days when the allergy symptoms appeared, but these bouts were fewer and less severe than she had suffered in the previous year. By the next season, the results were even more striking: in mold spore season, which was normally her most uncomfortable, she rarely needed any medication and was practically free of symptoms. Her experience with the allergy drops was a true success, enabling her to develop immunity and thus conquer her mold allergy.

For Carrie, traditional allergy injections weren't a viable strategy, since her sensitivity was so high that she could not tolerate dosages at the level needed to be effective. By contrast, even those people with very high sensitivity can tolerate allergy drops. Carrie and her scarecrow asthma brought home to me just how effective these drops are for chronic allergy sufferers—even those whom we once thought were beyond our reach.

Increased Air Pollution Makes It Hard to Breathe

It seems like common sense, but now we have proof. Recent studies have shown that ozone and nitrous oxide interact with airborne allergens to exacerbate asthma symptoms and increase the need for inhaler use. The findings in these studies showed that increased nasal mucus and wheezing were by-products of common air pollution (i.e., exposure to airborne allergens in the pollutants). And if that weren't bad enough, it also appears that some pollutants actually stimulate pollen production! Research shows that ragweed plants grow faster, flower earlier, and produce significantly greater amounts of pollen in urban locations, where the carbon dioxide concentrations and temperatures are *higher* than in rural locations. It also indicated that doubling the atmospheric carbon dioxide concentration *stimulated* ragweed production by 61 percent, which suggests that significant increases in allergenic pollen will occur in the future if global warming continues.[6]

Location! Location! Location!

Parents and allergy sufferers: pay attention to where you live! A recent study revealed that infants who live within 100 meters of "stop-and-go" traffic wheeze twice as often as those who live 400 meters away. Factors that increased this risk were the types of traffic and distance from home to the area of the heavy traffic. African Americans experienced the highest rate, at 25 percent.[7]

Home Is Where the Bugs Are

Indoor allergies are regarded as major culprits in the burgeoning allergy crisis. Newer homes that are more energy efficient and sealed tightly from the outside elements are breeding grounds for dust mites. Dust mites are microscopic organisms that you cannot see with your eyes but live in your household beddings and carpets. In fact, children lying on carpeted floors while playing Nintendo and Xbox for hours at a time are exposed to *billions* of dust mites.

It used to be that winter was the season when allergy sufferers found relief—no more tree pollen or ragweed to cause problems. However, what I'm now seeing each winter are more and more patients who come to the office complaining about a cold that won't go away. In most of these cases, they report no fever and the primary symptoms are nasal congestion and headaches. These patients suffer from "winter allergy" due to dust mites.

If you take your pillow and bang it against your mattress, you will see millions of tiny particles rise into the air and reflected in the sunlight. If these particles were placed under an electron microscope, you would see what looks like scary creatures right out of a sci-fi film. The good news is that, while disgusting, they're not infectious to you or others; the bad news is that we now recognize them as a major cause of indoor allergies that cause nasal and lung disease.

So if dust mites are around all year, why is this a winter allergy? The spike in dust mite allergy during the winter months is tied to the fact that in frigid weather, children and adults spend an average of less than twenty minutes outside each day—the remaining twenty-three hours are spent inside our homes, at work, or at school. For children, this means lying in their carpeted rooms (full of mites) and watching TV, or sleeping in beds with an entourage of stuffed animals (also full of mites). Dr. Thomas Platts-Mills at the

University of Virginia Medical College has done classic studies showing how children with greater exposure to dust mites were more prone to persistent asthma later in life.[8]

Heredity: Pass It On!

Simple genetics is another reason allergies are booming. Dr. Sally Wenzel, a noted allergy researcher, is fond of saying in her lectures, "Choose your parents well"—meaning, of course, your parents pass on their genetic traits, and unfortunately, this is also the case when it comes to allergies. If one parent is allergic and the other parent is nonallergic, their children have a 30 to 40 percent chance of developing allergies. If both parents are allergic, their children have a 70 percent chance of having allergies.[9]

Why have allergies been passed from one generation to the next? In evolution there must be some selective advantage for a trait to survive. But what is the advantage of the immune system having the ability to mount an allergic response? Some researchers have theorized that the eosinophil cells, those "forgotten" cells that we discussed earlier, and the allergic antibodies, IgE, may have been important to man's survival thousands of years ago. The eosinophils, for example, were important in fighting parasitic infections, which in the days before antibiotics and improved hygiene posed an ever-present and lethal threat to humankind. So eosinophils helped early humans adapt to their environment. It's a similar situation for IgE: It helped our ancestors fight parasitic infections.

Modern Medicine and Hygiene

One of the most surprising revelations about allergies is that modern medicine itself has contributed to their increased prevalence. How can that be? Modern medicine stands tall on its accomplishment of eradicating the deadly infectious diseases of humankind through drugs and vaccinations. In fact, vaccinations and antibiotics are what separated scientific medicine from quackery. It became clear that as modern medicine conquered infectious diseases, allergic diseases became more significant. So how can these monumental breakthroughs have made allergies worse?

Researchers have now been following epidemiological data that shows that allergies and asthma are more prevalent in developed Western countries than in Third World countries.[10] This truly has puzzled the researchers. Why is this true?

The "hygiene hypothesis" originally stated that the decrease in natural immunity to infections was due to vaccination and antibiotics, shifting the immune response to favor the development of allergies. But what was happening was that the natural immune response in children was not utilized by fighting the exposure to serious infections, so the immune system began to direct itself toward creating an immune response against allergens.[11]

Please Sneeze on My Child!

This was the tongue-in-cheek title of a *New England Journal of Medicine* editorial regarding the finding that children attending daycare in the first year of life were less likely to develop allergies and asthma than children not sent to daycare.[12] The researchers explained that children who attended daycare in the first year of life were exposed to more infections, which stimulated their immune system to become stronger at fighting infections and shifted the immune system away from developing allergies. This finding shocked the general public and perhaps made a few parents feel less guilty about sending their children off to a caregiver. Yet the same logic was applied to the finding that children with older siblings at home had fewer allergies; again, having more brothers and sisters increases the likelihood of exposure to infections, which strengthens the immune system to fight infections and shift away from developing allergies.[13] So you may not always get along with your brother or sister, but studies show that having them is good for you—if you want to keep from getting allergies.

Another befuddling find is that the past generation of children in the United States who have been vaccinated to mumps, measles, and rubella have seen these diseases eradicated;[14] yet this same generation is now being found to be more likely to develop allergies and asthma.[15]

Here's the final straw: playing in the dirt is good for allergies. A recent German study followed 812 children in Europe from rural areas, including those from both farming and nonfarming areas. Measuring a substance called *endotoxin* (which is found in dust and dirt) researchers found that the families with homes near farm animals had greater levels of endotoxin in dust from their mattresses and a decrease in allergies and asthma among their children. This important epidemiological finding is not yet fully understood, but it seems to indicate that endotoxin is a potent stimulator of the immune system and can help prevent the development of allergies.[16]

But what is a parent who has a child with allergies to do? Move to a farm? Allow dirt fights? Avoid vaccinations and antibiotics? Of course not! We have made so many strides in the last century with medications and vaccinations that have saved millions of lives. But as you'll read later on, we have many ways to "tweak" the immune system so that we can prevent and reverse allergies.

3

The Allergic Evaluation: It Doesn't Have to Hurt!

Here's a common scenario: a patient comes into my office, suffering terribly from sneezing, runny nose, itchy and watery eyes. She is petrified of needles, but I reassure her I can treat her allergies painlessly. I listen to her medical history. I examine her carefully. I take a sample of blood, which will tell me the specific cause of her allergy symptoms. The results show that she is allergic to her cat, as well as to pollens, molds, and dust. Based on this finding, I then have the information to make up a vaccine mixture, specially tailored to her particular combination of allergies, which she places under her tongue. She does this every day at home, and within a few months she begins to feel a great deal better, and after a year her symptoms have diminished considerably—or have vanished altogether.

Going to the allergist for testing today is a completely different experience than even just a few years ago. Once upon a time, a patient had to endure so many skin pricks to determine their sensitivities that many began to feel like human pincushions. No more. Great advancements have been made that make my job a lot easier, and my patients experience less anxiety and discomfort.

Many people fear the allergist, much like the dentist, because they believe they will experience unpleasantness and even pain. Because our preconceptions are often so far off the mark, in this chapter I will illustrate to you just how easy and painless it is to determine whether you are allergic—and to what.

Here are some of the most frequently asked questions that I hear from my patients:

Will it hurt?

Some of my adult patients recall going to the allergist as children and being placed on their belly to endure a hundred scratch tests on their back. That frightening experience scared them away from getting their allergies treated later in life and may also keep them from bringing their allergic children to be treated.

In place of the dozens of needles, a good allergist will come at you with dozens of questions. In fact, one of the most advanced tools we have for properly diagnosing allergy is very low tech: conversation. The allergic evaluation should begin with a careful history performed by a doctor, who will note the specifics about your symptoms to determine if an allergic cause is likely. Many of the questions will pertain to your current symptoms, but there also will be questions that seem unrelated but are equally important. A good allergist is adept at playing Sherlock Holmes, and the clue that often solves the case may appear in an unexpected place.

This all-important history taking will then be followed by a physical examination in order to narrow down the "suspects." Once your physician believes that the field is appropriately narrowed, the next step is to verify whether the allergy your doctor suspects is truly the culprit or causative factor in the complaints that have brought you in for testing.

Is there really a simple test?

Yes, testing for specific allergens is simpler than ever before. After I've taken the patient's history and performed the physical exam, all that's left to do is a simple blood analysis to determine the specific allergy antibodies. It really is that easy. In the past we required skin tests as well, hence all that prodding and poking with scratches. But today's sophisticated blood analysis allows for precise diagnosis with only one blood draw. The blood test tells us several important facts. First, it tells the physician generally how allergic a patient can be. This is called the *total IgE*. Much like knowing the number of your total cholesterol, for an allergic patient knowing his or her IgE is equally important. This test indicates the likelihood that the patient will develop, or has already developed, allergic antibodies to environmental substances (pollen, mold, dust) and foods.

For adults, any number over 114 is considered high, and any person with an IgE of 1,000 or more is highly likely to have an allergic disease. But just as with the total cholesterol, we know that one number is not the whole story; that is, there is good cholesterol (HDL) and bad cholesterol (LDL). Similarly, for allergic disease, knowing the total IgE is not enough. To make an accurate diagnosis we need what's called the *specific IgE*—an identification of the antibodies that are specific as to which allergens in the environment are the culprit. The specific IgE can reveal what you are allergic to and how severe it might be. For example, a high score of +4 to peanut may indicate you have a severe reaction to eating peanuts. This is a standardized test and very accurate.

What does my allergy score mean?

The new allergy blood tests are called the *third-generation tests,* because they are more advanced than earlier blood tests and a great deal more accurate. The *Pharmacia ImmunoCap* is an example of a highly sophisticated allergy test that can be easily interpreted by any physician. The scoring system is simple: the test assigns a number that tells you the degree of your sensitivity to a particular allergen. The higher the score, the more severe the allergy. To see how simple it is, just look at the chart that follows.

The scoring system is based on specific allergy units but translates into a simple scoring system for you and your doctor to review together. If you score a class 0 to all the different allergens tested, then you are most likely not allergic. A class 1 score is also very low and means you are also unlikely to be allergic, but you may need further allergy testing, such as a skin test, to investigate further. A class 2 score means you are allergic, but it may be mild or moderate. The class scores between 3 to 6 mean you have a significant allergy and that further testing is not necessary. A patient may possibly need a skin test if the clinical suspicion is very high and the blood test doesn't detect the allergen. The skin and blood do measure different IgE—one is bound to skin, the other is free floating in the blood.

Determining Your Allergy Score
Specific IgE Test Results, Clinical Correlations, and Management Options

Class	Specific IgE (kUA/L)	Levels of Antibodies	Clinical Correlation	Management Options
0	<0.35	Absent/undetectable	Consider nonallergic causes	Consider additional testing for infection or other diseases and treat nasal symptoms (decongestant)
I	0.36 – 0.59	Low	Uncertain clinical relevance; IgE antibody response may be a risk factor for future sensitization	Consider additional IgE testing in same category (e.g., trees) or as history suggests (e.g., foods, venom, drug)
II	0.60 – 3.49	Moderate	Probably a contributing factor to total allergic load	Consider additional IgE testing in same category. Consider implementing treatment options
III	3.50 – 17.49	High	Clinically relevant	Implement these treatment options: **For indoor allergens:** Institute environmental controls; If uncontrolled, trial of pharmacotherapy (OTC products, cromolyn, nonsedating antihistamines, intranasal corticosteroids, leukatriene receptor antagonist).
IV	17.50 – 49.99	Very High	Highly Clinically relevant	**For outdoor allergens:** Trial of pharmacotherapy (OTC products, cromolyn, nonsedating antihistamines, intranasal corticosteroids, leukatriene receptor antagonist).
V	50	Very High	Highly Clinically relevant	
VI	>100	Very High	Highly Clinically relevant	

Is the blood test as accurate as the skin tests?

This is a good question. All of the recent research indicates both types of testing are now highly accurate—close to 90 percent.[1] Since the two are equally reliable and accurate, I favor the blood test because it has two advantages: safety and standardization. Since you are not introducing the allergic substance into the body, there is no risk of an allergic reaction caused by the test. Also, the blood test is standardized (meaning the lab uses controls to make sure the test is accurate). Skin testing can vary depending on the device used and the practitioner performing and interpreting the test.[2]

For example, an allergy patient moves from California to New York to start a job. If she had the specific IgE ImmunoCap test done in California, she can bring these results in and I don't need to repeat the tests to treat her. The lab texts are standardized, meaning there is no difference from coast to coast! In addition, the blood test is not affected by medications like antihistamines. If your allergist is going to perform a skin test to detect allergies, you must discontinue use of all antihistamines for a minimum of forty-eight hours before testing. This could be a challenge for a patient who comes to my office in the middle of a terrible pollen season and is afraid to stop her medicine.

How specific can you get in these tests?

The testing can differentiate if you are allergic to cats versus dogs— or if you are allergic to fuzzy hamsters or not-so-cuddly mice. It can even tell you if you're allergic to horses. I have treated a few young men and women who were interested in becoming veterinarians and tested positive to many of these animals. I had to ask these bright young people to give careful consideration to their career choice, because their allergy test scores showed strong allergic antibodies to many animals, indicating a high likelihood of allergic symptoms if exposed to animals on a daily basis. I encouraged these students to go into "human" medicine instead of veterinary medicine. But one young man said, "I love the science of medicine, but I like that the animals don't complain!" Well, for him there's always the allergy drops.

Are some pets allergen free?

Most people who are allergic to dogs and cats react to animal dander—the dried, flaky material that animals shed from their skin. *There are no allergen-free cats or dogs,* but some breeds produce less dander than others, and in general *female* pets cause fewer allergic reactions than male pets.[3]

Veterinarian Marty Becker says the least-allergic dogs breeds are: small besenji, soft-coated wheaten terrier, bichon frise, poodle, Portuguese water dog, or mixed breeds like a labradoodle or other poodle mixes. The less-allergic cat breeds (and I say this with a tight jaw) are Cornish Rex, Dexon Rex, Siberian, or a sphynx (a mostly hairless breed). Dark-colored cats cause allergic reactions more frequently than lighter-colored cats.

Where can I get tested?

Today, you can get tested right in your own doctor's office. Pediatricians, primary care physicians, and internists all can order these allergy tests. Dr. Hugh Sampson, one of the world's leading allergy researchers, believes that it is critical for primary doctors, such as pediatricians, to start checking for allergies as a matter of course. He pointed out that 20 percent of the pediatric population is affected by allergies, and with all the advances made in testing, it makes good sense to have pediatricians screening for potential allergies.[4]

Studies have clearly demonstrated that allergy antibodies (IgE) to foods and airborne substances are highly indicative of more severe allergies and asthma in the future. In a key study, Dr. Alessandro Fiocchi, using a simple blood test, was able to determine which children were allergic, and to what. He found the test to be 93 percent predictive of which children were allergic and which were not.[5] (We'll discuss this in more detail later, but I must emphasize the importance of diagnosing children at a young age. Intervention and proper treatment can affect how allergies develop later in life and, in many cases, can greatly increase the likelihood of effective symptom management, or cause the allergies to subside completely.)

What happens if the blood test is inconclusive?

I will almost always screen a patient with the blood test first. If this gives me the information I need to conclusively determine the patient's allergy, then I don't do any further testing. Although the new blood tests are wonderful tools and have truly taken allergy testing into the twenty-first century, there are times when the results are not fully classifiable (+1) and it is prudent to do skin tests to support or rule out the allergen as significant. For example, if the blood test result comes back negative or very mild but I still strongly suspect an allergic cause, I will follow up with a few targeted skin tests in order to rule out the allergen entirely. If the skin test is also negative, then we can be almost certain the patient is not allergic, and occasionally the skin test will reveal a sensitivity that was not revealed in the blood test.

Today's skin tests are a great deal less painful and invasive than in the past. The device we now use is plastic and so quick, efficient, and painless that even toddlers are not generally bothered by it. Let me share with you the story of one of my patients: Lisa is a thirty-year-old woman who typically suffers from severe sneezing, runny nose, and watery eyes in the spring. This usually begins in April and lasts until June, when she finally gets a reprieve. She also notes that late in the fall she experiences shortness of breath and some wheezing that lasts for a few weeks. Lisa's blood test came back and showed these results:

Tree Pollen	+4
Grass Pollen	+4
Ragweed	+3
Alternaria Mold	+3

The test score showed a positive reaction (+4) to individual tree pollens and grass pollens. This is consistent with a very strong allergic reaction to these pollens and explains why Lisa's symptoms reoccur every year. She also tested positive to ragweed pollen (+3) and to Alternaria mold (+3). These two allergens dominate the fall months of September and October. With her history and these positive tests, I had a clear understanding of the specific triggers for her symptoms.

I hope I've dispelled the old myth in allergy that (just as in working out), "No pain, no gain." We see that allergy testing can be comprehensive, accurate, and accomplished in only one visit. Now we have to take that information and use it to protect you and win the battle against your allergies.

CHAPTER

4

What Are the Standard Treatments for Allergies and Asthma?

I n this chapter, we'll review the conventional treatments available for relief of allergy symptoms. It's essential to know what's available to you and the favorable and unfavorable aspects of each treatment. I believe that being an informed consumer is important and makes you a more active and engaged participant in your health care.

Participation is even more important when choosing medications. If you are working with a doctor who knows your medical history and is supervising your case, he or she is the ideal person to discuss your options with. Consider each option carefully, and do not hesitate to voice your queries and concerns—this is the only way to get the results you desire and to feel better.

For many of you, this overview will help you to better understand what has worked for you in the past, and what hasn't worked, and why. As we move forward in discussing sublingual allergy therapy, or allergy drops, and why this treatment offers the best options for treating your allergies or asthma, it is important to also discuss the medications that are commonly available and used. Most of all, what I hope to accomplish in this chapter is to help you see that a general pattern emerges when we speak about all of these commonly used medications—none of them is the silver bullet you are looking for.

Conventional treatments, while useful in the short term, and in particular contexts, are meant for occasional usage and are simply not the best long-term solution. To understand the inherent limitations of traditional treatments, we must distinguish between battling the symptoms of allergy, which some of these medications can do in the short term, and overcoming allergy for life, which none of these medications can promise. A review of the traditional therapies, including their individual strengths and shortcomings, is essential to arriving at an understanding of the breakthrough in allergy that will relegate all of these to a secondary tier. So let's begin.

Treatments for Allergies

There are a variety of conventional treatments for allergies. Each one is designed to alleviate symptoms, but may be suggested for different types of symptoms. Below is a listing of these medical treatments.

Antihistamines

For decades antihistamines have been the first line of treatment for all types of allergic reactions. It's an automatic: If you have an allergy, take Benedryl. Benedryl (its chemical name is diphenhydramine) is a well-stocked staple of every pharmacy, and you'll find it in almost every person's medicine cabinet at home—and most certainly in the households of anyone with a history of allergy.

This type of medication is extremely effective at controlling mild, acute allergic reactions, such as a spontaneous hivelike rash, a sneezing fit, or an itch in your throat. It is safe and effective and indispensable in a pinch, but is only a "quick fix." Its duration of action is limited to a few hours, and it only reverses the allergic reaction at a superficial level, which means it can't really resolve the problem, but it generally does hold it at bay for short periods of time.

Antihistamines are generally able to restore to you the upper hand when an acute allergic reaction strikes, but they are not able to relieve nasal congestion, a symptom frequently associated with allergy. In addition, there is a pronounced side effect to the older-generation antihistamines, such as Benedryl and Atarax, which is its sedative properties. Taking these medications will make you drowsy. In fact, recent studies show that these types of antihistamines not only cause symptoms of somnolence immediately, but they also have the latent effect of cognitive motor impairment, which means that a person who drives a car the day after using one of these medications will have slower reaction time when driving, and this can lead to accidents.

In an attempt to improve upon these classic antihistamines, the drug companies produced what is called the *first-generation antihistamines*. The names Seldane and Hismanal (both no longer on the market) and Claritin became top-selling medications. These drugs had the advantage of being *longer-acting* antihistamines, and even more importantly, they didn't usually cross the blood-brain barrier, which meant they wouldn't make you drowsy. When these medications hit the market, many in the field exclaimed, "Allergists better find another job. These medicines are wonder drugs. Who needs you guys?" But the elders in the field reminded us that the very same predictions were made when Benedryl first hit the market some sixty years ago. Two of the three "new and improved" antihistamines were removed from the drugstore shelves because they were found to cause a rare, but lethal, heart arrhythmia. The remaining medication, Claritin, did indeed become the top-selling antihistamine for a while, because it was found to be safe, and it had the benefit over the older medications of lasting longer and not causing sedation. Still, this was not the magic bullet.

The problem with all antihistamines is that patients develop tolerance to them, which means if you need to use the medication for weeks or months at a time (as many allergy sufferers do), your body builds up resistance to the medication, and it stops providing the same level of relief as it afforded you initially.

Challenges with Antihistamines

In my opinion, the real drawback with antihistamines is that they are more a Band-Aid treatment than a solution. Unlike antibiotics that eradicate infections, antihistamines don't and can't promise to give you lasting protection; they can merely ameliorate mild allergy symptoms. But no matter how well they suppress the symptoms, and no matter how long you keep taking them, once you stop the medications you are right back to where you started.

So as a doctor committed to healing my patients, the question on my mind is *what are you actually gaining?* I think antihistamines have their place, but as I explain to my patients, the key to long-lasting relief from allergies is to find and treat the underlying cause of the allergy—not just mask the symptoms.

In the meantime, pharmaceutical companies have been doing their best to engineer an antihistamine that truly delivers the relief that allergy sufferers crave, but this endeavor has its limitations. A serious concern with some antihistamines is the side effect of sedation. A study in 2002 showed that diphenhydramine (Bendedryl) impaired patients' ability to react quickly in tasks requiring cognitive-motor skills.[1,2] Antihistamines are powerless against nasal congestion and drug companies began to produce combination pills that contained both antihistamine and decongestant. So now your favorite antihistamines, such as Allegra-D, Claritin-D, and Zyrtec-D, were brought to market to solve all your allergy problems. Yet buyer beware: while these drugs may appear at first blush to be the answer to the dreams of allergy sufferers everywhere, they should be used only on a limited basis because of their possible side effects. Many of the patients who are referred to me by their personal physicians, for example, are people who have developed hypertension after prolonged use of such medications. Hypertension is a dangerous medical condition that can put you at risk for heart attack and stroke and can occur if you are taking these medications daily over a period of months. I've seen this occur even in young patients in their twenties and thirties who otherwise have no significant risk factor for hypertension. In addition, I tell patients with gastroesophageal reflux that they must try to avoid these medications. For these people, for whom excessive acid secretion is an issue, these medications can further aggravate the condition by increasing acidity and lowering the sphincter tone around the esophagus, allowing more of the acid to spill up into the throat. Yet another group of allergy sufferers who must be careful are patients taking antianxiety medications, because the decongestant contains properties that often make people feel "wired." In effect, the stimulant mechanism in the decongestant is working against the calming properties of antianxiety. In addition, many patients complain that the stimulant mechanism makes it difficult for them to fall asleep at night.

Hooked on Nasal Sprays

Kelly is a patient of mine whose story was a variation on the many I've heard from patients throughout the years. She started out with a cold that seemed to last longer than usual. A friend had recommended that she try this great over-the-counter nasal spray. Her friend took a bottle from her purse to show her and explained, "It will keep your nose open all the time." What the friend neglected to tell Kelly was that she carried that bottle of nasal spray with her everywhere because she had developed the need to use it every day to maintain that open breathing.

So Kelly took her friend's advice and started using the decongestant nose spray, and she was delighted with the results. She found it delightful that she could breathe easily through her nose once again. She, too, began to use the over-the-counter spray every day. Then one day on her way to work, Kelly forgot to put the nasal spray in her pocketbook. She didn't think about it again until lunchtime, when she realized she was very stuffy and couldn't breathe through her nose at all. She began to have a full-blown panic attack. She raced out of the office to the nearest pharmacy and bought a new bottle of nose spray, and right there she squirted it into her nose. Immediately, she felt relief. But as she calmed down, she realized that this didn't make sense. "I shouldn't have to depend on this little bottle *all* the time," she thought to herself. That's when she came to see me.

I immediately explained to Kelly that I could wean her off the nose spray by gradually replacing it with a nasal cortisone spray; the nasal cortisone spray wouldn't work as fast or be as strong as the one she'd been using, but she wouldn't become dependent on it, either. More important, I explained that if we figured out what was causing her nasal symptoms to occur in the first place, then maybe we could get her off nasal sprays altogether.

I took a detailed history and then, based on that information, I did some allergy tests that revealed that Kelly was allergic to her beloved cat. I outlined some options to remedy the situation, but she was very clear that Puma (her cat) was not leaving the premises. She asked what her *other* options were. I explained that when my patients won't remove their pet from the home, I suggest using the allergy drops to build immunity to the cat. Kelly was excited and said, "You can do that? Sign me up!"

We successfully got her off the nose spray to which she'd become dependent, and she used the nasal cortisone for a few weeks; then we were able to switch her to Nasalcrom, a safe, over-the-counter nasal spray that is not a decongestant and not a cortisone spray. Kelly also began the allergy drops, and within a few months she was feeling much better and no longer required any nasal spray on a regular basis.

Medications for Asthma

There are two main classes of asthma medication. The first are those I call "quick fixes," the medications that give you immediate relief by relaxing the muscles that have tightened to close the airways. These medications include the *beta-agonist* inhalers (Albuterol, which is the same as Proventil, Ventolin, and Maxair). The important point to remember is that these types of medications will give you instant relief, but they won't *cure* your asthma.

The other types of medication are critical to long-term control of asthma, and I call them the "mucus busters," because they can either break up the mucus in the bronchioles, or prevent its buildup. The "mucus busters" are either inhalers or pills that you take in your mouth; these include the inhalers Asmanex, Flovent, Pulmicort, Azmacort (these are inhaled cortisones, which are safer than oral steroids and many times help prevent the need for oral steroids). These inhalers are now more user-friendly and are not as difficult to use as they used to be.

There is also an inhaler that is a combination of both a bronchodilator (a drug that opens the airways) and mucus buster (inhaled cortisone) called Advair. It comes in a purple disc that looks like a little flying saucer and opens very easily like a camera. The delivery system into your mouth is very comfortable because it is breath-activated, meaning you don't have to pump it into your mouth; you just inhale and the medicine lightly goes through your mouth and down your windpipe into your lungs. It has many advantages in that it's a two-in-one drug—you only need one

---

Dangerous Decongestants

Decongestants, while effective in the short run, can be dangerous in the long run. Phenylpropanolamine (trade name Entex) was taken off the market a few years ago, because it was associated with increased risk of stroke in young women.

---

inhaler, not two. Asthma is known to be an inflammatory disease causing physical obstruction of the airways. It's important in cases of uncontrolled asthma to treat both components—inflammation and the obstruction—so that the inflammation resolves and stops producing mucus which narrows the airways. It also comes in different strengths, so dosage can be readjusted. I have found in my practice that prescribing the Advair discus has cut down my need to prescribe oral steroids by almost 75 percent.

Preventive Medicines for Asthma

Another category of asthma or anti-inflammatory medications is preventive medications. They are not indicated for an acute asthma attack, but are prescribed to try to keep asthma under control. The most popular of these medications is Singulair. It is a leukotriene antagonist and works to control airway inflammation in much the same way Ibuprofen does for muscle inflammation, but through a different biochemical pathway.

The other preventive medicine that many doctors seem to have forgotten about is Intal (sodium cromoglycate). It is based on the Mediterranean herb named Khellin and has been shown in many studies to help decrease symptoms if used forty-five minutes prior to exposure to an allergen. It is also approved for exercise-induced asthma and has helped a few Olympic athletes, such as Jackie Joyner-Kersee and Nancy Hogshead, on their way to gold medals. One challenge in prescribing Intal is that it doesn't work in about 40 percent of the patients. Those who successfully take it must be vigilant about regular use, because if you stop using the medication, you will relapse.

While we use the term *preventive* with asthma, it's not a literal use of the word, since it doesn't apply to preventing it from existing in the body—only from preventing attacks from occurring. Until I began using allergy drops in my practice, I was never able to provide a treatment that gave long-lasting protection.

Emergency Medicines for Asthma

There are several medications that are used primarily to control asthma symptoms once the condition has flared up. These are considered "emergency" medications and are solely for symptom relief. They are not effective long-term treatments and should not be utilized as such.

Corticosteroids

It is important to realize that corticosteroids (which are different from the androgenic steroids used in bodybuilding) were a major breakthrough in medicine in the 1950s to treat immune conditions like Addison's disease (President Kennedy suffered from this condition), as well as autoimmune diseases (where the body attacks itself), such as ulcerative colitis, multiple sclerosis, and allergic diseases. This was especially true for allergic asthma. This condition among children was thought to be a purely psychological disease. The use of corticosteroids changed the face of asthma—no longer were children confined to hospital wards for months at a time; in fact, asthma wards no longer exist.

Today, in most cases asthma can be managed at home or in a doctor's office. However, although steroids were a miracle cure for acute asthma, the use of this medication by injection or by pills on a chronic basis led to intolerable side effects: weight gain, osteoporosis (bone softening), cataracts and glaucoma, increased blood pressure, and increased blood sugar that could lead to diabetes.

With all the side effects of steroids, you are probably wondering, *Is the cure worse than the disease?* It was a tough choice for many doctors and their patients to make. The price for staying alive would be a poorer quality of life. Then came another ingenious breakthrough: *topical steroids*. Drug companies developed topical cortisone for the skin to treat conditions like eczema and psoriasis. They also developed topical inhaled cortisone for asthma and rhinitis. The beauty of the topical cortisone was that it blocked the allergic or immune reaction locally and without the side effects seen with the oral or injectable cortisone. These medications were a new weapon for allergists, dermatologists, and otolaryngologists (ENTs)—all of whom could now more safely treat their patients. ENT doctors, whose patients used to have to endure the pain of cortisone being injected into their noses, could now simply have the patients use a nasal spray. Dermatologists who had their patients covered in tar salves and oatmeal lotions could now use cortisone creams with quick relief and less mess. And allergists and pulmonologists could treat their asthma patients with effective inhalers that would reduce the inflammation in their asthma without the apparent side effects.

Monoclonal Anti-IgE: Xolair (Omalizumab)

This is a new hi-tech monoclonal antibody vaccine that has been approved for treating moderate to severe asthma. The concept behind it is that the anti-IgE binds to the circulating blood IgE, preventing it from binding to the surface of mast cells (boat cells) and basophils. While this description is certainly a mouthful, and may be difficult for the non-scientist or non-physician to fully grasp, in application Xolair is an exciting new therapy that shows promise in treating allergic asthma. I believe it is especially worth a try for patients who previously required daily oral corticosteroids.[3]

Again, these standard treatments, especially forms of cortisone, although widely used, have doctors all over the world wondering if they are safe for long-term use. The question is being hotly debated in many medical circles. Recent articles have raised the concern that even nasal sprays and inhalers that contain cortisone can cause osteoporosis, hypertension, and increased eye pressure when used over long periods of time, and in young children there is concern about bone growth. It is also important to remember that cortisone doesn't cure allergies; however, it can block inflammation by suppressing the action of eosinophils, T-cells, and other inflammatory chemicals produced by the body. Once these drugs are stopped, the symptoms can return if the allergic trigger is still there.

Medications are typically our best first line of defense in treating allergies, but the real goal is not to stifle the symptoms but rather to find the underlying cause of the allergy and then remove it so that it is no longer a constant source of exposure. That means that once the important detective work is completed and you've discovered the source of the allergy, whenever and wherever possible, the next step is to rid your environment of this offending allergen. So in addition to medications, the other traditional course of treatment is "cleanup."

Environmental Control and Avoidance

Once you've established immediate relief by medications, the next step is to try to remove or avoid the offending allergen—otherwise the need for medication will become chronic. Indoor allergens are well known to be a major factor in causing allergies and asthma. The problem is that people don't know the proper ways to rid their homes of the offending allergen(s).

Recently, a group of parents whose children had allergic asthma were surveyed to see whether they were taking the appropriate measures for environmental control in their homes. In four out of five cases, the parents reported at least one environmental trigger (animal hair, dust, smoke, mold, pollen) as the trigger for their child's asthma, and 81 percent of these parents attempted some action to remedy or remove it. Unfortunately, most of the actions taken by the parents turned out to be the wrong actions to take and did not help the situation.[4]

Dust Mites

The dust mite is the most common allergen found in the allergic population. Ninety percent of people with allergic rhinitis and 70 percent of asthmatics are sensitized to dust mites. Dust mites are living organisms that live off dead cells that we naturally shed from our skin as our cells die and are naturally replaced by newer cells. They thrive in humid environments and are mostly found in bedding, such as pillows, mattresses, box springs, comforters, and upholstered furniture. I have heard many stories over the years in my practice when a patient tests positive to dust mites: "Oh, my house is so clean. How can I be allergic to dust?" Or I hear the opposite: "Gee, I'm not really a good cleaner. I guess I'd better vacuum more often." The fact is that no matter how tidy you keep your home, you can't eliminate the dust mite, and more dusting and more sweeping won't do the trick.

To combat dust mites, some parents of allergic children put humidifiers in their bedrooms. This is completely counterproductive. The higher the humidity, the more dust mites thrive and proliferate. That's why dust mites don't survive well in cool, arid environments like Colorado or Switzerland. We all can't live in these places (as much as we might like to), but keeping the indoor humidity below 35 percent is a good start. This can be measured with the help of a simple, inexpensive device called a *hygrometer.* In fact, *dehumidifier* units and air conditioners, which lower humidity, can make your home less hospitable for dust mites.[5,6]

The overwhelming majority of dust mites are in your bed: on your covers, your linens, and the pillow. So in addition to sweeping and vacuuming, your best and first line of defense to reduce dust mite exposure is to encase your mattress, pillow cases, and box springs with specially designed impermeable covers that you can buy for precisely this purpose. For children, it is important to purchase stuffed animals and small cuddly toys that are machine washable so that you can routinely eliminate the dust mites.

Lastly, the heating in your home or apartment does matter. I see so many patients in New York who start to suffer with "the cold that won't go away" once the heat is turned on in their homes—usually in October or November. These "colds" are usually a result of dust mites circulating and blowing through heating vents. One possible solution if you have control of deciding what heating to use for your home is to consider radiant heating—unlike blowing vents, radiant heat doesn't kick up dust mites.

Don't Zap the Air

There are new concerns that the ionizing air cleaners advertised as good for you can actually be harmful, especially for people with allergies and asthma.

Ionizing air cleaners, also called *electrostatic precipitators,* are supposed to trap charged particles in the air. *Consumer Reports* initially evaluated these machines and found they did a poor job removing dust and smoke from the air. Now there is a bigger concern: these devices can be exposing you to significant amounts of ozone, which is particularly hazardous to people with allergies and asthma.

Ozone in the upper atmosphere protects us from harmful ultraviolet rays, but closer to the ground ozone can aggravate asthma. In the same study, the ozone was measured, and it was found that the level emitted was between 150 and 300 parts per billion (ppb), which is enough to cause significant problems for people with allergies and asthma. In fact, experts agree that ozone levels greater than 880 ppb for eight hours or longer can cause coughing, wheezing, chest pain, and worsening asthma. Such levels also make allergic people more sensitive to pollens, molds, and other respiratory irritants.[7]

Cat and Dog Allergy Management

It is estimated that over a third of the population has at least one cat in their home. That means animal exposure is high, whether you are coming into contact with your own pet or that of a friend, family, or neighbor. The cat allergen deserves special attention because it is highly potent. It is very light and can stay airborne for five to six hours at a time. That is why a person who is allergic to cats can go into a room and feel symptoms even if the cat is no longer present in the room. The cat dander sticks to walls, clothing, shoes, carpets, and furniture. Studies have shown that even after removing a cat from a home, residual cat allergen can still be measured several months later.[8]

Some of my patients are so allergic to pets that if they visit the home of a friend who has a cat, they immediately develop itching, sneezing, or experience difficulty breathing. They must immediately leave the house, because the symptoms quickly become intolerable. Even if the friend removes the cat from the main living quarters, the person usually still has symptoms, because the cat dander is in the form of very fine particles that remain airborne for days and months and are still being breathed in.

One story from my childhood left a lasting impression as to how severe and dangerous a cat allergy can be. When I was about thirteen years old, the brother of a good friend died. I later found out that he had experienced a fatal reaction to cat allergen: After a party, he had spent the night at his friend's house. The family had a cat, but put it in the basement for the night because he was so allergic. During the night, the cat snuck back upstairs and crawled underneath the bed where the boy was sleeping. He slept all through the night inhaling the cat dander, and in the morning he was found blue, having died from respiratory asphyxiation. The cat dander had caused his airways to close down.

This story truly has great meaning to me now as an allergist. I strongly advise my patients who are allergic to cats to avoid exposure when possible—but sometimes it's impossible. For these patients, allergy immunotherapy will not only improve their quality of life, but it can be lifesaving. I have used allergy drops to successfully treat many patients with cat or other animal-induced allergic reactions (dogs, horses, and birds), thus enabling them to be more protected and much less vulnerable.

Studies have recently shown that *HEPA filters* can reduce airborne cat allergen levels in the bedroom and living room, and this leads to reduced symptoms and improved respiratory function in patients with cat-induced asthma.[9] Another thing that you can do (while unpleasant for both you and your pet) is to wash your cat on a weekly basis. This has been shown to temporarily lower cat dander levels, but it has not been found to be an effective long-term solution.

The bottom line, however, is that it is very difficult to control or reduce animal dander exposure. The widespread distribution of cat and dog allergens was demonstrated in several studies that checked levels in schools and other public buildings. The researchers found high levels of cat and dog allergens in schools and on the clothing of schoolchildren. Notably, even children who didn't own pets were found to have significant levels of allergen on their clothes, which they brought into their own homes!

Managing the Roach Motel

I must admit that as an allergist one of my least favorite tasks is to break the news to a patient that he or she is allergic to cockroaches. Invariably the patient gets very defensive and is quick to speak of how clean his or her home is and the fact that they have never seen a cockroach where they live. How can they be allergic?

Well, these people are getting exposure somewhere. Most

cockroaches don't come out in daylight—if they do, that means there is major overcrowding in the "roach motel"—so many people may not even realize that these pests are living in their homes. Out of sight may mean they are out of mind, but the cockroach allergen is nevertheless present—sometimes in the walls and in tiny nooks and crannies, especially in many older homes. Their favorite locations are kitchens, bathrooms (they thirst for water), and bedding. They are a source of very potent allergens. Important studies done on inner-city asthma clearly link the cockroach along with dust mites and animal dander as important risk factors in asthma. Dr. David Rosenstreich of the Albert Einstein College of Medicine in New York City found that inner-city children with asthma were allergic to dust mites, cockroaches, and cats. The cockroach allergen levels in the bedroom of these children were five times higher than the dust mite and cat allergen. There is no mistake that the cockroach is an important indoor allergen. Children with cockroach allergy and high bedroom exposure levels were at a much greater risk for hospitalizations and urgent medical visits compared to children with asthma who were not sensitized to the cockroach.[10]

The control of cockroach infestation is possible, but it requires diligence. The basic idea is that to remove cockroach allergen, you have to remove the cockroaches. There are good pesticides that can accomplish this goal. However, before and after extermination, it is important to thoroughly wash and vacuum the home. Why do this? Even if you exterminate the insects, if food for them is available they won't go after the bait in the pesticides and they will come back. The key steps to prevent reinfestation are to seal cracks and holes, don't leave out dirty dishes or greasy pans, and keep leftover foods and dry cereals in sealed plastic containers.

Insecticides are your best chance for reducing cockroaches in the home. The organophosphates and carbamates have been around a long time and are generally 95 percent effective. A newer group of compounds called *avermectins* are odorless and also very effective. You can try to do the best job you can, but if you still don't get satisfactory results, consider using a licensed pest control company. They are allowed to use higher concentrations of the insecticides, are trained in safe application, and usually can improve the reduction of cockroaches in your home.

Dealing with a Mold or Mildew Problem

As mentioned in a previous chapter, mold is emerging as a bigger problem than ever before—probably due to climate changes. In addition to outdoor molds, mold is also a significant indoor allergen. Mold grows best in high moisture and humidity. I often hear stories from patients who say, "Gee, I always sneeze twenty times when I come out of the shower. Am I allergic to water?" Or the other classic history from a patient is: "Whenever I go down to my basement, I have difficulty breathing." The bathroom and basement are typically places of high moisture and humidity. Mold can take on many colors, from black to green to white. The major indoor mold allergens are *Aspergillus* and *Penicillium* (this is different than the medicine penicillin). The basic interventions are to remove the mold with fungicides that contain at least 10 percent chlorine bleach, to control humidity in basements with dehumidifiers, and to avoid vaporizers or humidifiers in the bedroom.

I can't stress enough how important it is to develop an environmental control plan with your doctor—or your children's doctor—so that you may undertake the appropriate interventions for your home, and in that way lessen your exposure or that of your loved ones. A very important multicenter study published in the *New England Journal of Medicine* by Dr. Wayne Morgan and Ellen Crain showed that a comprehensive environmental control program among inner-city kids with allergic asthma was as successful as medicine in controlling the children's asthma. The striking findings in this study were that 60 percent of the children's bedrooms had cockroach allergen on the floor and bed. Dust mites were found in 84 percent of the bedrooms. The majority of the children who had positive allergy tests to the cockroach and dust mites had detectable levels in their bedrooms. The researchers sent professional crews to eliminate the allergen. The crews were able to decrease the allergen levels by 50 percent, which translated into a significant reduction in asthma attacks among the children.[11]

While allergists generally urge their patients to implement environmental control and thereby minimize in their homes those allergens to which they are sensitive, compliance with these measures does not always follow. Studies have shown that *fewer than 50 percent* of patients adhere to environmental control—this includes the simple step of encasing mattresses and pillows to protect against dust mites and, of course, removing a pet from the home. And unfortunately, environmental control does not protect you when you visit the homes of friends and relatives where all these allergens may be thriving in the air. It's impractical to isolate yourself and impossible to live in a sterile, allergen-free world. So we should do the best we can to control our home environment, but since that can't protect us fully, I believe the answer is allergy immunotherapy, which enhances the body's own immune system to build a tolerance to what you are allergic to.

CHAPTER

5

The Concept of Allergy Immunotherapy

N ow that I've given you an overview of the conventional
allergy treatments and how they work, I'd like to focus your
attention on what I've been doing in my practice for the last few
years. Firsthand, I've experienced the first real groundbreaking
advance in the field of allergy in a long, long time—and one that
will forever change the course of allergy treatment. We are crossing
a new threshold and entering a new arena—one that allows us
finally to stop treating and to begin curing allergies.

Band-Aids versus the Solution

The difference between traditional allergy treatment and allergy
immunotherapy is not merely semantic and it will change the lives
of those with allergies. As you've just seen in the previous chapter,
traditional allergy treatments can go only so far in helping allergy

sufferers, because at best they are able to offer only transitory relief from the symptoms of allergy. Now we have the tools not only to quiet the symptoms, but also to reverse the underlying condition. What does this mean in practical terms for you and your loved ones who suffer from allergy? It means that we can now stop the coughing, sneezing, wheezing, and watery eyes by *reversing the allergic reaction itself.* In other words, lasting, lifetime relief is now available to you.

To fully appreciate the difference between treating the symptoms and curing the actual condition, consider the following example. Let's suppose that you are laid up with fever, chills, and a terrible cough due to a secondary infection, such as bronchitis, and that I gave you two aspirin. Within a short time, twenty minutes or so, you would likely feel better—and would continue to feel better *for the next few hours.* However, once those few hours passed, you'd be feeling just as wretched as you did before. The aspirin provides immediate and temporary relief of the symptoms, but it does nothing to address the underlying infection that makes you feel so bad. If, on the other hand, I started you on a course of antibiotics, although it might take a bit longer for the symptoms to lift, the relief would be lasting. The same principle applies with the newest allergy treatment: with allergy immunotherapy you now have at your fingertips an effective means to reverse the allergy itself—and a few drops a day is all it takes.

The Allergy Solution

Sublingual allergy immunotherapy, or "allergy drops," is a natural and convenient way to assist your immune system in building up its own tolerance to the allergen(s) causing your symptoms. Using your immune system as a barrier to allergens is the optimal solution for long-lasting results. This breakthrough treatment, which has been used successfully in Europe for many years, is now available here in the United States in liquid drop form that can be placed under the tongue. The treatment is safe, simple to use in the convenience of your own home, and proven to be effective. It must be prescribed by a physician who will target your specific allergies through this vaccine.

I have enjoyed the extraordinary privilege of seeing remarkable improvement in my patients as a result of this allergy therapy, and their renewed vitality is the greatest advertisement for it. Even the worst allergy cases will see dramatic improvement, and the sufferers' lives will be transformed. Each time I have personally overseen an immunotherapy treatment, the improvement has far exceeded the expectations of the patient, who has been used to using medications and sprays to temporarily relieve their symptoms. People whose allergies previously crippled them or kept them from enjoying many of life's activities were able for the first time to lead a normal life: play golf without a box of Kleenex, go over there friend's barbecue who has a cat. Others who had dealt with the irritation of chronic symptoms were amazed and delighted to discover how sweet life became once they were liberated—for good.

How Allergy Immunotherapy Works

The mechanism behind allergy immunotherapy is simple and elegant, and you don't need to have a degree in science to appreciate the mechanism. The treatment is analogous to lifting weights. We all know that working out is good for us, but the only way to get stronger is to lift more weight. The more often we do so, the stronger we become and the more efficiently our bodies operate. Similarly, in allergy immunotherapy, a person's immune system builds up protective blocking antibodies when the patient receives gradual, stronger doses of allergy drops. The stimulation to the immune system creates a shift in the immune balance to block allergy symptoms instead of developing such symptoms.

The beauty of allergy drops versus injections is that you are getting small, safe doses daily, but at the same time your body is getting a quantity of medication that is one hundred times higher, which leads to immune protection. Typically, a patient's starting dose will be exponentially small, about the amount of particles if a cat shed one hair on you. But through the process of increasing the concentration of the drops every month, eventually you would be taking a dose equivalent to the cat's full coat, but would no longer have symptoms.

I've always found that in learning science a picture is worth a thousand words, so I've included an illustration here to show how allergy drops help your body develop immunity against an allergen. The diagram (Concept of Immunotherapy) shows two pathways: (1) how allergic inflammation occurs, and (2) how protective immunity develops.

The picture at the top shows an allergen (a cat hair, or a pollen grain) symbolized by *a speckled baseball* binding to the IgE receptor (the "black Y") on the mast cell. This "little catch" between the allergen and the IgE receptor determines if allergic inflammation, meaning an allergy attack, will take place. IgE receptors are adjacent to one another and have "caught" an allergen, and then the TH2 cell will release chemical messengers (cytokines IL-4, IL-5) to cause an allergic reaction. To block an allergic reaction, as in immunotherapy, the TH1 response is favored and blocking IgG antibodies are made, which inhibits the allergic reaction.[1]

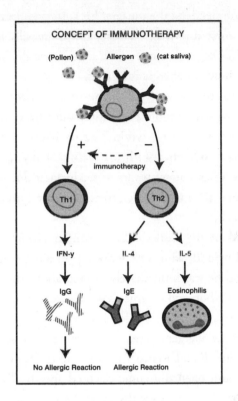

Where Did This Treatment Come From?

The concept of allergy immunotherapy in this country dates back to the 1920s, when Dr. Robert Cooke, who was an attending doctor at New York Hospital, became interested in this subject. Dr. Cooke was highly motivated because he was himself a very allergic person. Specifically he was allergic to animal dander, including horsehair, which posed quite a problem for him back in the 1920s, when horse and buggy was still the primary mode of transportation. During his internship he was bedeviled with allergic reactions and asthma but at first didn't understand the cause of his suffering. In those days, he was riding a horse-drawn ambulance, and eventually he recognized the pattern and began to understand that it was the horse that was the culprit behind his allergic reactions.

The only treatment available at the time was adrenalin. So Dr. Cooke was busy self-administering adrenalin injections so he could continue to function in his work. The problem with adrenalin is that it has many side effects—heart racing, shaky hands—not the type of things a sick patient wants to see in their doctor. Dr. Cooke was determined to find a better treatment for himself and other allergy sufferers.

He learned of the work of Dr. Leonard Noon and Dr. John Freeman in England, who were working on allergy desensitization to pollens, and he was immediately excited about this research. Dr. Cooke studied Noon and Freeman's work carefully and then extrapolated information from it to develop new allergy treatments for different airborne allergens based on the same premise. He was then able to treat himself and eventually moved to the Roosevelt Hospital in New York and opened a clinic devoted specifically to the diagnosis and treatment of allergic diseases.[2]

Building on the work of these predecessors, Dr. Cooke pioneered the work of allergy immunotherapy at the Roosevelt Hospital. He successfully came up with injection regimens to treat adults and children who suffered from hay fever and asthma caused by pollens, animal dander, and house dust. This work was further refined years later by doctors at Johns Hopkins when Drs. Philip S. Norman, Lawrence M. Lichtenstein, and Peter Creticos demonstrated that its success could not be written off as mere placebo effect and showed what dosages were critical to making immunotherapy effective.

The Roots of Oral Allergy Immunotherapy

The initial use of an oral allergy treatment dates back in the medical literature to the late 1800's. A tincture of fresh flowers made from "ambrose" was used to treat hay fever. In the early 1900's, Dr. Curtis tried flower and pollen vaccine from the fluids of ragweed taken by mouth—with good results. In 1927, Dr. Black demonstrated that large doses of oral ragweed extract worked in decreasing nasal symptoms. In 1919, Dr. Schamberg used drops made from a tincture of *Rhus toxicodendrum* (poison ivy), which was found to be useful in rural areas of the United States to prevent park workers from developing poison ivy.[3] The limiting factor on these treatments was that the large quantity of allergen ingested caused digestive problems: mouth irritation and dyspepsia. With the advent of sterile instruments, the use of injections became the technical advancement that left the oral method in the dark for almost half a century. Interest in an oral form of allergy immunotherapy was resurrected by French and Italian researchers who made a technical adjustment to the way oral immunotherapy was to be given—under the tongue (sublingual route). In the 1970's, Dr. David Morris, working in relative obscurity in the small town of La Crosse, Wisconsin began treating patients suffering with allergic rhinitis and asthma with sublingual allergy drops. Almost twenty years later, in 1998, Cutis published his article on using sublingual allergy immunotherapy to treat nickel dermatitis. The door was starting to slowly open to oral immunotherapy, but it would still have a long way to go.

The concept of allergy immunotherapy is that the immune system can be taught not to overreact. With immunotherapy you start with the tiniest doses and expose the patient to the very allergen he or she is allergic to, and then very gradually build up to higher and higher doses until the patient's body builds a tolerance to the allergen. By building a tolerance to the allergen, the immune system is learning to tolerate and to stop overreacting to what should be a harmless substance. The patient's system is challenged with higher doses to evoke the immune system to better tolerate and not overreact to what should be a harmless substance.

The beauty of this therapy is that it truly is a natural: you are receiving a substance that you are allergic to and allowing your immune system to solve the problem. Unlike a drug, which is a foreign substance to the body that has to be broken down in the liver or kidney and can cause side effects, immunotherapy doesn't interact with other medications. It has a history of being safely used in pregnancy and has not been found to be teratogenic (causing harm to an unborn fetus) as some drugs can be.

How I Came to Discover Sublingual Allergy Immunotherapy

One day in the spring of 1998, an event transpired that left me determined to find a better solution to the problem of allergies. Every allergist knows the risk associated with allergy injections, but when you actually live through the experience with a patient, that is a whole other matter. I'd like to share the story of what happened that day and how it led me to the discovery that a "secret" cure already existed, one that was truly the answer to my prayers—and the prayers of allergy sufferers everywhere.

On the day in question, I had just finished a very busy day of seeing sixty patients. It had been an unusually warm spring day, and patients were suffering terribly from their allergies. That entire spring was particularly bad for patients who were sensitive to pollens and molds, and this was an especially tough day for these people. At the time I had been in private practice for more than seven years, and, like every allergist, I treated many of my patients who suffered from severe allergy with allergy shots.

A young woman named Jill came to my office late on this day for her routine allergy shot. Jill was receiving weekly injections for pollens and molds. And although allergy injections are for the most part extremely safe, the process quickly delivers the allergen into the bloodstream, which can trigger a potent allergic reaction and carries the risk of a severe, or *anaphylactic*, response. Within five minutes of her injection she began to feel flushing all over her body and was sweating and having difficulty breathing. I realized immediately that she was having an allergic reaction to the injection and gave her another injection containing adrenalin to try to reverse this reaction. The adrenalin did decrease some of her symptoms, but it also caused her to have palpitations and extra heartbeats. I knew this was a potentially dangerous situation, so we called 911, and I went with her to the hospital to be treated and observed until her heartbeat became normal.

Jill had experienced what allergists call a *systemic reaction;* this is where the body is overactivated by an injection of allergy vaccine and the body releases massive amounts of histamine. These reactions can be severe and even fatal. Dr. Richard Lockey, a professor of allergy and immunology at the James Haley Veterans Hospital in Tampa, Florida, is an expert on fatalities due to allergy injections and has written guidelines to warn physicians about the risks involved when allergy injections are given. However, even Dr. Lockey notes that a fatal reaction can occur even if everything is done properly.

That evening, I was emotionally and physically drained from what I had seen Jill go through. I was attempting to treat my patient's allergies, but she could have died from the treatment. When I got home, I hit the books with a whole new resolve, determined to unlock the key to finding a better way to treat my patients. Usually it is only in the movies that we are treated to one of those pure Hollywood moments, when the music swells and sheer determination and grit are rewarded in the blink of an eye. Well, that night I enjoyed a real-life moment of such uncanny and surreal good fortune. As I was reading through the most recent professional journals, I came upon an issue of *Cutis,* a respected journal for allergists and dermatologists. My attention was immediately riveted upon an article that presented the option of using immunotherapy, but without the shots.[4] This seemed too good to be true and would defy all the common wisdom in the field. The article outlined an alternative method of delivering the allergy vaccine to patients—rather than administering a shot, you simply placed the vaccine under the tongue. I was incredulous at first. Drops instead of shots? It seemed impossible: I had never heard of this, even though I kept up with the literature and attended most major allergy seminars. If it hadn't been published in such a reputable journal, I might have dismissed it as quackery—and perhaps if I hadn't been as motivated by the day's events, I might have passed it over. As it was, I was enthralled by the article and the promise it posed.

Learning from the Best

Dr. David Morris was the author of the article, and he was presenting a case report of allergy sublingual immunotherapy to treat nickel allergic contact dermatitis (a condition similar to poison ivy, only with nickel it generally comes from jewelry or metal buttons on pants, or brassieres).[5] Morris's idea was fascinating, but what was truly exciting to me was the fact that he included references at the end of the article about sublingual immunotherapy to airborne, environmental allergens. That meant the treatment might also work on those patients who were sensitive to pollen and mold, like Jill! I was so excited that my heart was literally pounding. Could it be true that you could get the full benefit of allergy shots (immunotherapy) without the shot? If that was truly possible, then why had I never heard about it? For an allergist, a discovery like this was probably similar to discovering the lifesaving properties of antibiotics or the vaccine for polio.

With my enthusiasm unabated, I found Dr. Morris's name and phone number in my medical directory for allergists and called him first thing in the morning. Once I identified myself and gave the reason for my call, Dr. Morris explained that he was really surprised by my call and also surprised that the article had appeared in the medical journal *Cutis*. I was confused by his response until he explained that he had submitted that article fifteen years ago and had long ago assumed they would never publish it. Dr. Morris went on to say that he'd been a tireless crusader for this new treatment for many years, and that he'd attempted to share the results of his work with academic allergists at a variety of respected institutions, but his message seemed to fall on deaf ears. "Too controversial for the guys in the ivory towers," he concluded, but he was delighted that *Cutis* had finally decided to publish the article and to discover that someone else was interested in this work. He invited me to visit him at his office and see firsthand how this therapy worked.

At the earliest opportunity I flew to Wisconsin to meet with Dr. Morris to learn more about his allergy drops and to see for myself whether this new treatment was too good to be true. As I drove by the beautiful farmlands that stretched out as far as the eye could see, I had a lot of time to wonder whether I'd gotten carried away by the events that transpired with Jill, and whether I was deluding myself into believing in fairy tales. In the course of that drive I wondered why Dr. Morris's work had received such a cold shoulder for so long a time. My collective conscious came up with different thoughts: "old treatments die a slow death in medicine," or the "tried-and-true treatments" don't fall easily by the wayside. This has always been the hallmark of conventional medicine. It is of course why people trust doctors and medicine: the white coats, the prescription pads—these are what many patients are used to and comfortable with. Anything new is met with resistance, and the medical community must be won over to try it. Ironically, sometimes the push for change comes from the public.

When I arrived in La Crosse, Wisconsin, I met with Dr. Morris at his office, which was an old converted schoolhouse. Dr. Morris was a kind-looking man and spoke with a soft and deliberate accent. We sat down in his consultation room, and he told me how he had started out as a family practitioner, delivering babies and performing appendectomies. He was the type of old-fashioned "doc" that America revered. After a stint in the air force, he decided to focus in allergy and initially treated patients with allergy injections. But he, too, found that patients would sometimes have severe adverse reactions from the shots, and, being inquisitive, he was always on the lookout for new treatments. (He chuckled when he told me he was the first doctor in his community to have a cardiac defibrillator and that the other doctors thought he was crazy to be "shocking patients' hearts" with arrhythmia. Now, of course, we know cardiac defibrillators are standard treatment for cardiac arrhythmias.)

He told me about his journey to Europe, where he met with a young Italian allergist-researcher named Walter Canonica. In his office in Italy, Dr. Canonica pulled out stacks of research papers published in European journals showing the effectiveness of sublingual allergy immunotherapy. "I knew I was onto something," Dr. Morris smiled.

Dr. Morris then showed me around his office facility. It was very impressive and had large waiting rooms for three other doctors. There was a large laboratory where allergy tests were performed on blood samples from patients. He told me that together he and his three colleagues saw over a hundred patients a day and that people traveled from all over the Midwest to see them—from Iowa, Minneapolis, and other remote towns—almost all word-of-mouth referrals from patients who had been treated successfully.

It was music to my ears to hear, straight from Dr. Morris, that in more than thirty years of using sublingual immunotherapy he had never had a patient experience severe allergic reaction from the drops—like the one I had recently experienced with my patient Jill in response to the allergy injection. Yet he also reported that the drops were consistently effective over a broad spectrum of patients—and he'd been using this treatment for thirty years, which meant he'd had extensive clinical experience with the drops. But I was even more impressed when I saw the evidence with my own eyes as I observed Dr. Morris treating his patients: sublingual allergy immunotherapy reversed allergies.

No More Shots! Sublingual Allergy Immunotherapy

After visiting with Dr. Morris and viewing this brave new path for allergy treatment, I was determined to follow in his pioneering footsteps. Injection immunotherapy was a flawed but promising form of treatment—and one that deserves to be reformulated rather than discarded. That is precisely what has been accomplished in the groundbreaking treatment of sublingual allergy immunotherapy. The principle behind why the sublingual treatment works is exactly the same as with the more traditional injection therapy, but instead of being administered through shots, the sublingual treatment is given through oral drops, placed under the tongue.

The truth is allergy shots were the most effective form of treatment we had, because they addressed the allergic response itself, not just the symptoms. The problem was the delivery system—injecting the vaccine—inevitably carries the risk of an anaphylactic response.[1]

Making allergy immunotherapy into an orally administered treatment makes more sense because of the safety factor. So why hadn't anyone thought of this before, and why had no one heard of it? After all, the idea has precedent: the reason we rarely administer penicillin by injection these days is precisely because of the rare but possible deadly allergic reaction. Instead, and as a rule, we give penicillin orally.

The idea to give a treatment sublingually may, at first glance, seem strange. Who would think of giving a medicine under the tongue? But for decades doctors have prescribed nitroglycerin sublingually to alleviate chest pain. The sublingual route takes advantage of direct absorption (but in a slower fashion than an injection) into the venous bloodstream through the *mucosa* (tissue) under the tongue. The medicine or, in this case, allergen is absorbed without being destroyed by the enzymes in the stomach.

The concept of oral immunity even predates modern medicine. Native Americans discovered on their own that tribesmen who licked the leaves from poison ivy were less likely to develop reactions to later contact with it, or if they did, the reactions were significantly less severe.[2]

It wasn't until the 1980s and 1990s that researchers, primarily in Europe, began to take another look and to investigate in earnest the notion of sublingual allergy immunotherapy. It was the French and Italian researchers who led the way—exploring the possibility that you could successfully immunize a patient for allergies by giving them allergy drops. A number of researchers, like Drs. Jean Bousquet, Andre Clavel, and Walter Canonica, began to have successful results by placing the allergy extract under the tongue and having the patient hold it there for two minutes and then swallowing it.[3, 4]

What was the magic in having the patient hold the liquid extract under the tongue instead of just swallowing it? The researchers realized the importance of the absorption of the allergen under the tongue into the rich, lymphatic tissue there.[5] The lymph tissue took in the allergen and presented it to the rest of the immune system so that it could get used to it and not overreact in such a way that mimicked a severe natural allergic reaction. After many positive studies, it was demonstrated that sublingual swallow of allergy extracts were also effective against dust mites, pollens, and molds.

By the late 1990s there were numerous studies that show the benefit of sublingual-swallow allergy immunotherapy. In November 1998 the World Health Organization (WHO) had its meeting on *biological vaccines* (this is the new term for allergy extract). Their report stated, "Well-designed studies employing high dose sublingual-swallow immunotherapy provide evidence that this form of therapy may be a viable alternative to injection therapy in the treatment of allergic airway disease."[6]

The more I researched, the more evidence I discovered in support of this treatment, so it became all the more confounding that there was such a resounding silence on the subject—at least in the United States. In trying to figure out the cause for this disconnect, I determined that there were a number of possible reasons that contributed to the explanation for this highly effective therapy failing to get its well-deserved recognition. First, the research being done on sublingual-swallow allergy immunotherapy was almost exclusively done in Europe and published in European medical journals, and sometimes it takes longer for science to travel across the Atlantic.

While Europe was focusing attention on this new vaccine, here in the United States new research was focused almost exclusively on finding new allergy pharmaceuticals. Why? In part this can be explained by economics—after all, the pharmaceutical companies have tremendous resources and are able to provide a seemingly infinite stream of research dollars. Compared to the major pharmaceutical manufacturers, those that make allergy extracts (vaccines) are much smaller and don't have that type of funding.

Following in the Pioneering Footsteps of Dr. Morris

I returned from La Crosse, Wisconsin to my practice in New York, excited yet nervous about beginning this new form of treatment. When you are going against the grain, the isolation surrounding you can raise nagging doubts. *Does it really work? Is it safe?*

I reminded myself that Dr. Morris had been practicing this therapy for thirty years without incident, and also that the medical literature clearly supported sublingual therapy as both safe and effective. Ultimately for me, I found the more frightening prospect was the idea that I might shy away from this new frontier and continue with the traditional path only to have another patient endure a severe and potentially life-threatening allergic reaction to an allergy shot. It was one thing to take that risk in the past, but to do so now, when I knowingly had the choice to offer a safer and equally effective alternative to my patient, was unthinkable.

Dr. Morris had given me detailed instructions on how to start a *rush protocol* (This is an accelerated way to reach high doses in a short time period.) to get started in my practice. I also called two of the top allergy programs in the country: Johns Hopkins and National Jewish Medical Center. I explained to the research allergist what I planned to do. Both were familiar with the European work on sublingual-swallow immunotherapy and said that as long as proper protocol was followed they saw no reason why it wasn't reasonable to try.

The two main criteria that motivated me to change from shots to drops were safety and efficacy—meaning *were the drops safer than shots with regard to serious allergic reactions? and did they work?* Two fine papers published in Euorpean allergy journals clearly answered these questions.

Dr. Claude Andre in France looked at the safety of the sublingual-swallow immunotherapy in children and adults. He reviewed 690 patients, including 472 adults and 218 children, who received allergy drops to various allergens: grass and tree pollens and dust mites. Dr. Andre and his group reviewed patients on sublingual-swallow immunotherapy (SLIT) for four months to two years. Their review found mild reactions in some of the patients: oral itching and some gastrointestinal symptoms, but *overall no serious adverse events were reported!*[7]

Taking it a step futher, Dr. V. Feliziani from Italy did a rush study of allergy drops to grass pollen. He looked at thirty-four patients with rhinoconjunctivitis (nasal and eye allergies) with or without asthma. The patients receiving allergy drops showed a reduction of symptoms of rhinoconjunctivitis and asthma and a lower intake of medications—all statistically significant! No patients showed local (meaning in the mouth or stomach) or general side effects! These studies gave me the green light I needed, and there was no turning back.[8]

Now it was my turn, I instructed my staff on the proper way to make up the new dilutions of allergy vaccine that would be needed to treat my patients who suffer from ragweed pollen—a condition we typically refer to as hay fever—in August and September. When we were preparing the solution for the patients, we placed the solution in a dropper vial so that the patient could accurately place the correct number of drops under his or her tongue.

The patients in my practice who were allergic to ragweed were given the choice of whether to be treated with allergy medications or to try this new sublingual immunotherapy. Thirty patients opted for this new type of treatment. I instructed the patients on this rush protocol, explaining when and how many drops they were to take each day, and told them they were to complete their treatment and stop administering the drops by August 15—the onset of the ragweed pollen season.

All of the patients completed the month of drop therapy without any problems. This was important to me, as it gave me confidence that this route of therapy was safe. The question now was whether it would prove to be as effective as medications or the allergy injections. Because it was mid-July by the time I got the treatment organized it was a treatment of short duration; ideally it would have been better to begin these patients on the drops for a longer period prior to the ragweed exposure. It was hard to gauge the success of this initial round of treatments. The majority of my patients felt there had been a reduction in their allergy symptoms after using the sublingual vaccine. But I still wanted to see if I could improve and refine the treatment to demonstrate without equivocation that this treatment was effective.

Rush Immunotherapy

Several years after I began offering to my patients the opportunity to use allergy drops, a large, multicenter clinical trial was performed in Canada studying ragweed pollen. Ragweed has long been known to spoil the end of the summer for millions of allergy sufferers on the East Coast—for these people, Labor Day barbeques and picnics are nothing to look forward to, because the pollen usually peaks during this time.

The Canadian researchers followed 57 patients. The active treatment group (28) received allergy drops to ragweed pollen, and the placebo group had 29 participants. The unique aspect of rush immunotherapy is that the patient's doses were rapidly increased to high dose levels over a seventeen-day period, while the usual protocol is to stretch that out over several months. The first four days they received low doses, then for the next four days the dose was increased tenfold, and finally the dose reached a maintenance dose three times stronger. This dose was given throughout the entire ragweed season. The results were exciting: the patients receiving the ragweed sublingual allergy immunotherapy (allergy drops) had fewer symptoms during the season, and their blood tests showed that they developed higher protective allergy antibodies (IgG).[9] This was the first study in North America showing the effectiveness of the allergy drops, and specifically to a significant allergen—ragweed.

No More Shots

Josh is a fourteen-year-old boy who is a terrific soccer player. He is a starting forward on his middle school's soccer team. After a day of playing hard, Josh and his mother both noticed that he would develop puffy eyes, sneezing, and coughing. They brought him to my office to be evaluated, and I found that he was highly allergic to tree and grass pollen. This clearly explained his eyes, nose, and chest symptoms. Josh's symptoms were particularly bad in the spring on the lush grass soccer fields. He had tried over-the-counter antihistamines, but they made him too tired to keep up with the other players. He had also tried the newer antihistamines, but they weren't strong enough to control his symptoms. I recommended immunotherapy to Josh and his mother. The mother said, "Thanks, but no thanks." A few years earlier, Josh had seen another allergist who had recommended allergy shots. Josh hated getting the needles, and his mother hated schlepping him every week to the doctor's office. After a short time, they just stopped going.

I informed both of them that we now had a new option, sublingual allergy immunotherapy, which meant Josh could now take drops at home to prevent his allergies to trees and grasses. I saw big smiles come across both of their faces. Josh said, "Are you serious? No more shots!" I nodded, as delighted to provide this welcome news as they were to hear it. Then his mother asked, "And we don't have to come every week for these drops to be given in the office?" I told her that Josh would be responsible for taking them at home each day. "Sign us up," she said.

Josh self-administered his drops in the sublingual allergy immunotherapy for a full year and reached good maintenance doses. His symptoms to the tree and grass pollen decreased significantly, and now he is finally able to go full speed for the entire duration of his soccer games.

I found Josh's situation to be a case in point for why sublingual therapy is advantageous over injection therapy: patient compliance. When the patient hates getting shots every week and the mother hates bringing him to the allergist's office every week, the likelihood of the patient reaching maintenance levels and successfully completing the treatment are low. The beauty of the sublingual therapy is that it is done at home by patients, and at their convenience. Both the adult and pediatric patients under my care have reminded me of how truly disciplined patients will be when you give them some control over their treatment. I've found that the compliance rate among my sublingual immunotherapy patients who are reaching maintenance levels is an extraordinarily high 97 percent. By contrast, researchers have found that the compliance rate among those receiving allergy injections and are reaching maintenance doses is less than 30 percent.

Sublingual allergy immunotherapy has become such a successful component of my practice that I have all but ceased administering allergy injections, as have many of my colleagues. Ask your doctor or allergist about allergy drops, or visit www.AllergyChoices.com for listings of physicians that administer allergy drops in your area.

How Long Until I Feel Better?

The common question patients ask me is, "When will I see improvement?" My experience with patients has demonstrated that symptoms usually began to decrease in the first year, but in the second and third year, symptoms significantly decreased.

Dr. M. Marogna, an Italian researcher, and his group showed objective evidence that sublingual allergy immunotherapy not only decreased symptoms but also improved breathing function in patients with allergic asthma and decreased the eosinophils on nasal smears in patients with allergic rhinitis.[10]

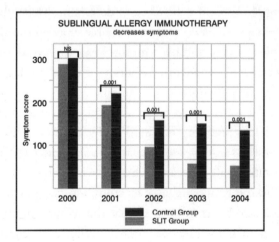

The bar graph is easy to follow: the gray bars represent the allergy patients receiving the allergy drops, and the black bar represents the allergy patients receiving traditional medications. In year 2000, before patients got into the active study, the symptoms scores were the same. By 2002, the patients on the allergy drops showed significant reduction in symptoms compared to the medication group. In addition, the allergy drops showed objective measures of improvement: stronger breathing tests and fewer eosinophils on nasal tissue. So the big question is: when will you feel better? Be patient. During the first year of treatment, you should feel noticeably better. But, by the second year you should not only feel *even better*, but allergic parameters will also show that you *are* indeed better by a medical definition.

The Protocol of Sublingual Allergy Immunotherapy

The protocol for sublingual allergy immunotherapy is very simple. First, allergy testing must be done to determine what substances a patient is allergic to. If the patient is unable to avoid the allergen or has multiple allergens and his symptoms extend beyond one season (meaning a chronic problem), a dilution of the allergen goes into a dropper vial to be used under the tongue.

The patient is instructed by my medical staff on the first visit of therapy to place one drop of liquid under the tongue and hold it there for thirty seconds. Holding the liquid under the tongue is extremely important, because this is where the allergen gets absorbed by the lymph tissue. The studies in the past where oral therapy failed to benefit indicated that the subjects didn't hold the liquid under their tongues; they either swallowed it completely or spat it out.

The Oldest Medical Caveat: Do No Harm

Safety, as I mentioned earlier, was what first attracted me to the concept of allergy drops. Initially I was relying on Dr. Morris's thirty-year clinical experience treating more than one hundred thousand patients—and that's certainly not anything to scoff at. However, the medical literature has clearly supported this view, as numerous studies have shown the safety of the treatment even in young children. Up until recently most allergy practice guidelines in Europe and the United States have advised against starting immunotherapy for children under the age of five. The main concern within this age group was safety—such young children can't always adequately voice adverse reactions.

A new study looked at the safety of allergy drops in children aged three to seven years and found there was no difference in reactions to the medication between these young children and older children, and therefore there was no need for this particular treatment to be withheld based on age. The argument for treating these young children is that in the first five years, many children exhibit the symptoms of the "allergy march" in skin rashes such as eczema, and studies I will discuss later show that diagnosing and treating allergies when children are young can stop the "allergic march" so that there is no progression in sinus disease and asthma.

Patients are instructed not to eat or drink for thirty minutes after taking the drops. The reason for this is that we don't want any interference with absorption of the drops through the lymph tissue. The majority of patients take their drops after they brush their teeth in the morning or the evening. This seems to work because the patients develop a routine, which is key to long-term compliance.

It is also recommended that the patient use a handheld mirror so she can see exactly how many drops are going under her tongue. When I first started prescribing the allergy drops, I watched my patients as they self-administered their drops and noticed that a great many patients misjudged what they thought was one drop; oftentimes it tended to actually be several. The patient was observed in the office, and if there was no reaction, they were instructed to increase to two drops the next day and then to four drops on the third day. They were to continue the four-drop regimen daily for an entire month and then return to receive either a stronger dilution or to add more allergens.

It is also important to review with the patient at the outset the possible adverse reactions that can occur with any medical treatment. The sublingual treatment is much safer than the injections, but it is still possible to experience itching in the mouth, a rash, or swelling. If any of these reactions occur, I tell them to take oral Benedryl and to call my office for further instructions on dosing changes. I've had a rare one or two patients develop a rash, but this was resolved with antihistamines. I also caution the patient about possible respiratory reactions to the drops, like shortness of breath or wheezing, although this is rare. The cornerstone of this treatment is that patients receive increasingly higher concentrated dilutions so that they can build a protective, lasting immunity. That is the trick to doing any immunotherapy. With immunotherapy we are "working out" your immune system to build up tolerance to what you are allergic to; this is done by challenging the immune system with a low dose of allergen and gradually building up to increasingly high doses, which will give lasting immunity.

The real advantage of sublingual allergy therapy is that it is a custom-tailored treatment for each patient. Unlike drugs, or even herbs, allergy drops are specific to each patient. Herbs and drugs target the body's chemistry to block a biochemical reaction in the body. They are not specific for the particular allergen; instead, it's "one size fits all." In allergy immunotherapy, however, we make a specific allergy vaccine to allow the body's immune system to develop protection to the allergen and make a vaccine that is specific for each patient. Researchers are hoping in the future to make cancer vaccines with the same concept—"designer vaccines" that are specific for the individual patients with cancer.

Allergy Therapy Shouldn't Feel Like a Prison Sentence

Instead of weekly visits for allergy shots, the patient needs to receive monthly vaccines. That means vacations or travel for work will no longer mean an interruption in therapy.

A study by Dr. Canonica showed that objective findings occurred in the second year of treatment with patients who had allergic asthma. They found improved breathing tests and nasal smears that showed fewer eosinophils from these patients, which are associated with allergic mucus.[11]

Why do allergy drops work so great? Because my patients use them regularly. My practice and the medical literature support the evidence that 90 percent of patients on sublingual allergy immunotherapy are compliant (meaning they don't miss) with their treatment.[12] This is in sharp contrast to allergy injections where the compliance is around 30 to 40 percent.[13–16]

As an allergist I am also familiar with the considerable tension that can occur when one person in the family unit is diagnosed as being allergic to the pet and the others are not allergic. This is likely to stir up tension in the family when the allergic patient's symptoms are relatively mild. When a loved one is in serious or obvious distress (severe wheezing or trouble breathing, for instance), the other family members are more responsive. Some of my patients, upon chronic exposure to the cat dander, will eventually begin to notice they have constant nasal congestion—"the cold that never goes away"—or they become more susceptible to sinus infections due to decreased nasal drainage. In some cases, the patients develop a chronic cough that can lead to asthma.

Jeff's Story

One such case was particularly memorable. Jeff was forty-three years old, worked as a pharmacist, and was in peak health. He was an avid tennis and basketball player and had a youthful look about him. However, on one particular visit to my office he didn't look anything like the man I knew. He had a swollen face as a result of gaining fifteen pounds, and he looked depressed.

Jeff began explaining that he had just been released from the hospital two weeks earlier, after a severe asthma attack. He had never had asthma before. He recalled some chest congestion and shortness of breath a few weeks before his hospitalization, but he attributed these symptoms to a lingering bronchitis from a few weeks before. He still continued his weekly tennis matches and pickup basketball games, but he noticed his stamina was decreased. Then came the point three weeks earlier when he woke up in his bed and could barely catch his breath. He panicked and called his primary care physician, who gave him a breathing treatment to open his lungs. He felt slightly better and was given a prescription for an inhaler and steroid pills to hasten his recovery. However, a few days passed and Jeff wasn't improving. His doctor recommended he go into the hospital to get oxygen and intravenous steroids. After five days in the hospital, Jeff's breathing was less congested, but he was extremely lethargic from all the medication. He was moody and depressed, and he hated relying on inhalers to keep his lungs open. Jeff came to my office, desperate to find out why this happened.

After listening to Jeff's story, I took a detailed history of any possible new exposures to allergens at his home or work. I questioned him about possible reactions he may be having to substances at the pharmacy where he worked mixing chemicals or drugs. He told me he didn't do that anymore. Another pharmacist performed those functions. Jeff was now mainly involved on the business end. I asked him if there were any pets at home. He looked at me quizzically and said, "Yes, why does that matter?" I explained that people can be allergic to their pets and not even realize it. He then mentioned that his wife had brought home a cat about three months ago. He didn't care much for the cat, but his wife loved it and was frequently bringing it into the bedroom to sleep in their bed with them at night. He did also notice that during these past few months he felt congested in his nose and chest when he awoke in the morning and that his symptoms got better as the day went on while he was at work.

I told Jeff that I was concerned he might be allergic to the cat and that we should perform some allergy tests to determine if this was the case and, if so, how severe the allergy was. The allergy testing showed that Jeff was highly allergic to cat dander. On his weary face, I now saw a smile. He finally had an answer as to what was causing his problem. He thanked me for my time and assured me that the cat would be removed from his home. Before he left, I wrote some prescriptions for inhalers to control his breathing until he fully recovered.

Two weeks later I got a call from Jeff. He needed to see me urgently. I was concerned that his health had taken a turn for the worse. I wondered, *Did I miss something in the diagnosis?*

Jeff returned for his next visit looking healthier than I expected, and he was accompanied by his wife, Erica. They walked into my exam room and both thanked me again for my help in getting Jeff better. Once we were in the room, Erica took control of the conversation and Jeff remained quiet. She couldn't believe that her precious little kitten was the cause of Jeff's asthma. She had never heard of such a thing. I tried to explain to Erica that cat dander was a highly allergic substance to certain people and that from my testing of him, I was quite certain that Jeff was one of these people. Her disbelief began to turn to anger. She asked, "Well, isn't there anything that can be done?" I explained that removing the cat was the best option. She responded unflinchingly, "No, I mean aren't there any treatments for this cat allergy?" I explained that allergy immunotherapy could decrease a person's allergic sensitivity to cats. She smiled upon hearing this news and said, "Great, then he'll do it." I said I thought it was important that they discussed this option privately between themselves and that Jeff could get back to me if he wanted to do the treatment. Jeff had been silent the whole time.

One week later he was back in my office. He said, "Let's begin the allergy immunotherapy. My wife made it clear—I'm going before the cat is!" I treated Jeff with the sublingual allergy immunotherapy, and he improved over the course of the year. He never had a severe asthma attack again.

How Do I Know If It's Working?

I monitor patients on the sublingual allergy immunotherapy by scheduling appointments with them a few times during the course of the year. I want to make sure, first of all, that they are compliant with the therapy. This also allows me to track their progress. I have patients fill out questionnaires regarding their health, any new medications they are taking, and the time they are to receive their next dose of drops. In the first year of the buildup phase (raising the allergy doses in the drops)—usually in about six months—patients will notice fewer symptoms to the substances they are allergic to. If they are allergic to cats, for example, in the past they might immediately sneeze or wheeze when being around cats. After several months of allergy drops, the symptoms would be less severe and take longer to appear. If they are allergic to grass, ragweed, or tree pollen, they should notice less need for medication, and while their coworkers are sneezing and miserable at the beginning of the allergy season, the people on allergy drops might not notice symptoms until the end of the season.

How Long Do I Continue Taking My Allergy Drops?

The question of how long allergy immunotherapy should be administered was a mystery for almost seventy years. The data available on that question was too flawed to draw any reliable conclusions. In the past, if you went to an allergist he was likely to tell you that if you required allergy shots, you would need to continue getting those shots for life. The assumption was that the protection offered to patients through these shots would disappear unless you repeated the treatment weekly for life.

Dr. Stephen Durham, a highly respected allergy researcher in England, published an important study in the *New England Journal of Medicine* that showed that people receiving allergy injections at a maintenance dose for three years did no better with an additional three years of treatment than patients who also received the same treatment for three years and then received a placebo (water injection).[17] This seemed to imply that after three years, patients on allergy immunotherapy had received the maximum benefit and that further injections were unnecessary. In other words, the current thinking is that you need to continue taking the treatment until you've reached your maximum protection level. Once you've hit your maximum level (after two or three years in most instances), the protection is considered lasting.

In the next chapter, Dr. Canonica's studies show that after three years of sublingual allergy immunotherapy patients with allergic asthma were significantly less symptomatic and needed less medication—and seven years later were still allergy and asthma free.

If you have been impressed by what the allergy drops can do for hay fever, wait until you see it's affects on asthma.

CHAPTER

7

The Asthma Action Plan

O ver the last two decades the number of asthma cases in the United States has quadrupled—a change for the worse that has perplexed doctors and scientists. Advancements in medical science have enabled us to do so much to thwart other illnesses, like heart disease, but even though we have effective medications at hand and are able to effectively *treat* the growing numbers of asthma cases presenting, the problem is that we are seeing more and more new asthma sufferers. There are many competing theories about why this increase is occurring. While there is no definitive answer as yet, I personally believe that the increasing asthma morbidity is in large measure due to environmental factors, and that many doctors are overlooking the important connection between allergies and asthma. Once you acknowledge the allergy-asthma connection, the increase in the incidence of asthma becomes less bewildering, though no less troubling. I have devised an Asthma Action Plan to empower you to take control of your asthma with your doctor. I believe in the maxim: "Give a person a fish, and he will eat for a day, teach a person to fish and he will eat for a lifetime." It takes discipline and persistence to become cured from asthma—but it's worth it.

The Asthma Action Plan has three phases: (1) a control phase, (2) a reversal phase, and (3) a prevention phase. But first you have to understand asthma.

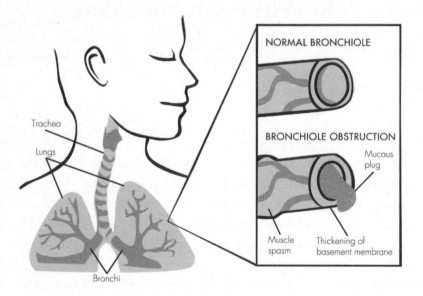

What Is Asthma?

Asthma is by definition a *reversible* blockage of the airways in the lungs. During an asthma attack the airways become inflamed, which means the lining becomes swollen and narrows the cavity through which air can pass. That narrowing is what makes breathing difficult. The narrowing can reverse, sometimes by itself, or other times with the help of medicine. When asthma is present, the lungs are supersensitive and often constrict when exposed to a spectrum of different allergens, irritants, or changes in weather.[1]

The symptoms you are likely to experience with asthma may include a feeling of tightness in the chest, shortness of breath, wheezing, or a dry cough that lasts more than a week. The triggers of asthma have been known for many years. The things that most commonly set off an asthma attack are environmental allergens, irritants, infections, stress, and sometimes food. In the past the infections and stress triggers got most of the attention. If the trigger was an infection like a secondary bronchitis following a cold or virus, the solution or remedy was readily apparent: administer antibiotics and a bronchodilator such as Albuterol. If the trigger was extreme stress or the fact that the person had not developed adequate coping tools to handle stress, then once again the remedy was clear: see a therapist. Years ago, if a child came into a doctor's office wheezing and short of breath, the doctor would automatically prescribe antibiotics and a bronchodilator. However, we now know that this one-size-fits-all approach is not good enough. Asthma is an inflammatory disease, and while antibiotics can clear the infection that may have been a contributing trigger, they cannot clean up the resulting mucus and chemical secretions from the lungs, and as long as those substances are there, the lungs will remain constricted. Until you address all the effects caused after the original triggering incident, you are not fully treating the patient.

Control Phase

To effectively treat your asthma, the first thing you have to know is to what degree it is out of control. Surveys have shown that most young adults with asthma are unaware of its severity or how much it compromises their lives. People with asthma begin to accommodate their discomfort. For example, it was not unusual for adolescents with uncontrolled asthma to wake up several times during the night and use their inhaler—never telling their parents; they thought this was normal.

The Asthma Action Control Test is a quick screening method to give you an idea if you need to better control your asthma.[2] Answer each question below and write that answer's number in the box to the right of the question. Please answer as honestly as possible. This will help you and your doctor discuss your asthma treatment plan and determine whether your asthma is controlled as well as it could be.

1. In the past four weeks, how frequently did your asthma keep you from getting much done at work, school, or at home?

All of the time	Most of the time	Some of the time	A little of the time	None of the time
1	2	3	4	5

2. During the past four weeks, how often have you had shortness of breath?

More than once a day	Once a day	3 to 6 times a day	Once or twice a week	Not at all
1	2	3	4	5

3. During the past four weeks, how often did your asthma symptoms (wheezing, coughing, shortness of breath, chest tightness, or pain) wake you up at night or earlier than usual in the morning?

4 or more nights	2 or 3 nights a week	Once or twice a week	Once a week	Not at all
1	2	3	4	5

4. During the past four weeks, how often have you used your rescue inhaler or nebulizer medication (such as Albuterol)?

3 or more times per day	1 or 2 times per day	2 or 3 times per week	Once a week or less	Not at all
1	2	3	4	5

5. How would you rate your asthma control during the past four weeks?

Not controlled at all	Poorly controlled	Somewhat controlled	Well controled	Completely controlled
1	2	3	4	5

Add up the numbers that correspond to your answers, and write your total score in the box shown.

If you scored 19 or less, this suggests your asthma may not be under good control. In general, the higher you score, the better your control. The ideal score is 25.

Once you are aware of your asthma's severity, how can you assess your breathing? A simple instrument called a *peak flow meter* measures how well you move air through your lungs. Peak flow meter readings monitor asthma in much the same way that blood pressure readings help a patient monitor hypertension. Relatively inexpensive, the meter costs about twenty dollars and can be purchased at any local pharmacy. A peak flow meter is an extremely valuable tool for assessing your breathing and helps you understand if your asthma is worsening and in need of medical attention.

A peak flow meter is a device that measures how well air moves out of your lungs. The peak flow meter is used to detect narrowing in the airways hours, even days, before you have any symptoms of asthma. A peak flow meter can help you decide when to stop medication or add medication based on the readings. It alerts you when to call your doctor or seek emergency care. You can feel confident that your asthma is being accurately monitored. And most important, it can help you communicate with your doctor.

How to Use a Peak Flow Meter

Your peak flow should be measured before you use your inhaler (preferably at 8:00 in the morning and between 3:00 and 5:00 in the afternoon). Timing is critical in interpreting long-term peak flow numbers. Of course, if you are worried about your breathing, you can use it anytime to determine whether you need to adjust the dose of your medications or call your doctor.

1. Place the Best Effort indicator at the base of the numbered scale.
2. Stand up . . . Take a deep breath.
3. Place the meter in your mouth and close your lips tightly around the mouthpiece. DO NOT block the opening with your tongue.
4. In ONE breath, blow out as *hard* and *fast* as you can!
5. Write down the number the Best Effort indicator reaches.

Repeat the above steps two more times and try to get a higher reading.

Understanding Your Peak Flow Meter

To regulate your asthma more closely, we break down the reading into three categories.

1. Your Excellent Zone—This is 80 to 100 percent of your predicted best score.
2. Your Careful Zone—This is 50 to 80 percent in your predicted best score.
3. Your Danger Zone—This is less than 50 percent of your best readings.

These zones are calculated based on your age and height. And will be part of your written Asthma Action Plan.

Self-Assessment

1. What was your highest score? _____
2. What time of the day did you score the highest?
   8:00 AM   5:00 PM (circle one)
3. Do you find that keeping track of your peak flow readings makes you more aware of whether your asthma is really good or bad today?
   Yes   No   (circle one)

Asthma Action Plan

It is essential that you have a written plan to manage your asthma. The National Institutes of Health recommends that every asthmatic patient should develop such a plan in conjunction with their physician.[3] The Asthma Action Plan lets you understand how well controlled your asthma is and whether you need more or less medicine. If your asthma is worsening with symptoms such as wheezing, chest tightness, or shortness of breath and your peak flow levels are low, you may be in the danger zone. Immediate interaction with strong medications like oral cortisone may reverse this severity of the asthma and help you avoid ending up in the hospital. Following is a template of your Asthma Zone Grid. The medications should be decided between you and your doctor. Martin Mongone, now chief of respiratory therapy at Beth Israel Medical Center in New York, and I have successfully used these tools in seminars teaching patients with asthma how to be more proactive in controlling their asthma.

Asthma Zone Grid

Level 1: Excellent Zone: This happens when your breathing is under good control and near your best.

Peak Flow (80–100 percent) ____
Your medications should be:

_____ inhaler _____ puffs at ____ AM ____ PM ____ PM.
_____ inhaler_____ puffs at ____ AM ____ PM ____ PM.
_____ pills _____ mg at ____ AM ____ PM ____ PM.

Level 2: Careful Zone: This can happen when you catch a cold and you feel chest tightness, shortness of breath, or wheezing. Also, remember chronic coughing can mean your breathing is getting worse. If these things happen, your peak flow may drop and require an adjustment in medication.

Peak Flow (50–80 percent) ____
Your medications should now be: (Order is important: bronchodilator first and mucus breaker second)

_____ inhaler _____ puffs at ____ AM ____ PM ____ PM.
_____ inhaler _____ puffs at ____ AM ____ PM ____ PM.
_____ pills _____ mg at ____ AM ____ PM ____ PM.

Level 3: Danger Zone: This happens when you are having a lot of trouble breathing and are not responding to all the above medications. If your peak flow is below 50 percent, you should start taking prednisone according to your instructions and call your doctor. Prednisone should be taken with some food, and please tell your doctor if you have gastrointestinal problems or other medical conditions (such as depression) so that your medication can be adjusted properly.

Peak Flow (less than 50 percent) ____
Your medications should now include all the inhalers from level 2 (Careful Zone) plus:

_____ pills/liquid_____ mg at ____ AM ____ PM.

Once you stabilize your asthma, the Asthma Action Plan helps you and your physician judge if you are at a higher level of breathing and can use less-potent medications.

I have trained many of my patients to become aware when they are moving from the excellent to the careful zone because of a cold or allergen exposure. By adjusting your medications quickly, we can avoid more discomfort and get you back to normal.

As an example, I'll tell you about a patient I'll call Derek. He came to my office after being referred by a friend because he was short of breath and wheezing. Derek's condition seemed especially bad during changes of seasons or when he developed a cold. He was using his Albuterol inhaler indiscriminately, sometimes four times a day, and on other occasions up to eight times a day. He didn't realize he was using a "quick-fix" inhaler without the help of a "mucus buster."

I wrote up an Asthma Action Plan for him based on his age, height, and symptoms to determine his asthma management zones. Since he was symptomatic and his peak flow was initially 350 (careful zone), I had him start on a combination of a bronchodilator and a mucus buster. Advair 100/50 twice a day achieves this with one inhaler. Derek dutifully recorded his peak flows every morning before he used his inhaler and again before using his inhaler in the evening. After five days he noticed that his peak flows were rising and his wheezing and shortness of breath were abating. After two weeks his peak flows had risen to 560 and he was symptom-free. I then explained to him that we could switch him to an Intal inhaler twice a day. (He was now in a condition to use this nonsteroid inhaler because his breathing was in the excellant zone.)

The zone system is a highly efficient way to monitor patients with asthma, and any patient with asthma should ask his or her doctor to write a plan for home use. And work with your doctor to find out the finer points to keep your asthma under excellent control.

HOW TO USE AN INHALER

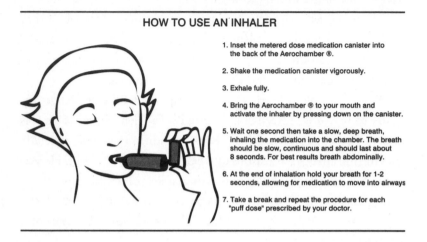

1. Inset the metered dose medication canister into the back of the Aerochamber ®.

2. Shake the medication canister vigorously.

3. Exhale fully.

4. Bring the Aerochamber ® to your mouth and activate the inhaler by pressing down on the canister.

5. Wait one second then take a slow, deep breath, inhaling the medication into the chamber. The breath should be slow, continuous and should last about 8 seconds. For best results breath abdominally.

6. At the end of inhalation hold your breath for 1-2 seconds, allowing for medication to move into airways

7. Take a break and repeat the procedure for each "puff dose" prescribed by your doctor.

If you use a *metered dose inhaler* (MDI), I strongly recommend you purchase a chamber device, which makes it easier to inhale your medication and get the full dose. If you have a dry powder device, the holding chamber is unnecessary.

Examples of Mistakes

With MDIs

- Failure to shake the inhaler well
- Failure to exhale slowly before inhaling

Examples of errors with MDI spacer devices

- Placement of inhaler in the wrong end of the spacer
- Failure to first exhale slowly
- Failure to shake inhaler well

Example of errors with dry powder inhalers

- Shaking the inhaler
- Failure to first exhale slowly
- Exhaling into the device (this can result in clumping the powder)

> ## A Need to Clear the Air
>
> The safety of using a the long-acting beta-agonists (Serevent) Salmeterol and (Foradil) Formoderol have come under intense scrutiny.[5] The danger of using these bronchodilators alone, which open the airways and give people relief, is that in most cases they need an anti-inflammatory medication such as an inhaled steroid, oral steroids, or a leukotriene antagonist (Singulair), because bronchodilators (beta-agonists) don't combat the inflammation in the bronchiole walls. So the beta-agonist opens the airways for a set time, but doesn't clear the garbage (the mucus). As a result, it's like a garbage truck's compactor door opening and shutting down, but the garbage keeps piling up. For a patient with asthma this means the airways get plugged up and air can't pass through.

Using a metered dose inhaler is not as easy as it looks. If you ever watched someone else do it and they look like they're doing a "hit" of Binaca the breath freshener, then you know they are doing it wrong. An inhaler should be done in a deliberate way and below are the common errors made by patients.[4]

Reversal Phase

Once your asthma has been medically controlled with drugs, the next step is to reverse the inflammatory component of your asthma at a deeper level. Today the medical literature clearly supports the link between allergens as a cause of the inflammatory component of asthma. In my mind there is absolutely no question that in many cases allergy is the trigger that sets asthma in motion. Unfortunately, many patients with asthma have no idea they are allergic and have never seen an allergist, so the primary trigger for their condition is going untreated. That is why I call the association between allergy and asthma "the lost connection." I remember speaking to an old-time family practitioner who was greatly respected in the community. He had come to attend a lecture I was giving on asthma around the same time that he was getting ready to retire. After the lecture he came up to me and said, "You know, Dr. Mitchell, I think my generation missed the boat on the importance of allergies as a cause of asthma." I truly respected this doctor, because he was one of the few who had the courage to see things from a new perspective after a lifetime of practicing in a different way.

I believe the key to reversing asthma is treating the patient's underlying environmental allergies by sublingual allergy immunotherapy. It works at the deep level of the immune system to build up protection from the inflammation caused by the allergen. I have seen time and time again where a patient has a cat and over time develops asthma. It has been gratifying to reverse the patient's asthma by treating their cat allergy with sublingual allergy immunotherapy. The patients developed a tolerance to the cat dander and no longer needed their asthma inhaler. The same is true for pollen allergies. Let's look at Mark's story.

A Treatment That's Easy to Swallow

Ten-year-old Mark is one of my patients. He has light brown skin, dark brown eyes, straight black hair, and a grin that spreads from ear to ear when you talk to him about baseball. Mark speaks in a high-pitched nasal voice, but is very articulate and poised for someone of his years. During my first office visit with Mark, his mother, Maria, was visibly upset when her son dejectedly explained that he couldn't play Little League baseball in the spring. Mark had fallen in love with America's favorite pastime. He loved scooping up ground balls and running the bases. His secret dream was to be a major league player. However, during the preceding spring baseball season his asthma and allergies had become intolerable. After being on the field for a few innings, Mark's eyes would become watery and swell up. He would also experience difficulty breathing. He'd have to come off the field between innings to get extra puffs of his asthma inhaler, Albuterol. After these games Mark would be up all night coughing and wheezing, and his mother would have to hook him up to his home nebulizer and give him several treatments before dawn. Mark's pediatrician tried to manage his allergies with antihistamines, like Claritin, and his asthma with inhaled cortisone, but it just didn't seem to do the job.

Mark came to see me because a relative who knew me recommended he visit my office for an evaluation. When Mark first told me his story and confided his secret, I told him we had something in common—I had been an aspiring baseball pitcher, too. My problem wasn't allergies however, but the fact that opposing hitters started creaming my fastballs! Mark broke into a smile, and I could tell I had his trust. I did a complete medical history and then examined him. When I listened to his chest, musical noises emanated from inside. It sounded like an accordion opening and closing.

I told Mark and his mom that I was confident I could help him. First, I would draw some blood to test for specific environmental allergies. It was clear to me that tree and grass pollen played a major role in triggering his symptoms, but I wanted to be determine precisely how severe these symptoms were and also determine whether any other less obvious allergens were also contributing to his problems. Mark and his mom agreed to the tests, and I did the blood work, telling them that I expected to have some answers for him in a week. In the meantime, we would control his symptoms with a combination of inhaled cortisone and a bronchodilator inhaler.

Mark returned the next week feeling slightly better and very curious to know what he was allergic to. I took out a piece of paper from the lab that listed all the allergy tests performed on Mark. The highest scores were to trees, grasses, and ragweed, but he was also allergic to dust mites and animal dander (dogs and cats). We discussed our options: using daily medications every spring, trying the allergy drops, or no more baseball. Mark and his mom felt medications weren't doing the job. The no-more-baseball option was definitely not a choice they wanted to make. Then they looked at each other and smiled. The allergy drops were their best hope and they wanted to try it. We started Mark's treatment that fall. By the time spring came around, he had had about six months of allergy drop treatment. He went out for Little League, and this time there were no more time-outs for itchy, watery eyes and no more quick breaks for his asthma inhaler. The allergy drops had already begun to build his immunity to the outdoor pollens and helped keep Mark symptom free. Dr. Steve Salvatore, the medical correspondent at New York City's Fox 5 News heard about Mark's story and came to the office to interview him. Dr. Steve was impressed with Mark's story, but since it was a warm summer day and Central Park is just around the corner from my office, he couldn't resist an outing to see if Mark's results were too good to be true. The two of them set off with some baseball gloves and tossed the ball back and forth in the park's ball fields. Dr. Steve came away a believer. When he aired the interview, he gave it the title "A Treatment That's Easy to Swallow."

Can We Reverse Allergic Asthma Once It Already Exists?

As in Mark's case, the latest research suggests that allergy drops can reverse asthma. Dr. Walter Canonica is one of the leading allergy experts in the world. A recent past president of the World Allergy Organization, he has done much of the initial research that has brought sublingual allergy immunotherapy to mainstream academic and clinical allergists.

Dr. Walter Canonica's groundbreaking study showed that treatment with allergy drops can not only decrease symptoms and

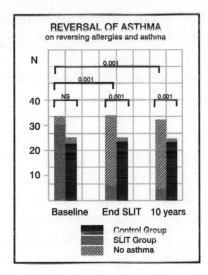

the need for medications in patients with allergic asthma, but they can also help to *essentially reverse the asthma into remission.*[6] The study was done with children with allergic asthma who had positive allergy tests to dust mites. It has long been established that dust mites are a trigger and cause asthma in allergic children. The children in the study were assigned to either a control group receiving placebo or an experimental group receiving allergy drops to dust mites. The results, as shown in the figure above, were striking.

If you look at the two bars labeled baseline, SLIT (allergy drops) versus CTRL (sugar-water drops, the control substance), you see the two groups of children with allergic asthma. The dark gray portion indicates active asthma, meaning the children were symptomatic and required medications to control their symptoms. The light gray portion of the bar indicates subjects who were free of asthma symptoms. Initially, both groups had very little light gray, meaning that all these children were symptomatic.

Now let's look at the data from the time after both groups had completed their treatments, three years later. (Remember, in this double-blind study one group was actually taking the allergy drops, while the other was only taking a sugar-water placebo.) Do you see the stark contrast emerging between these groups? Three years out, those who took the real allergy drops showed a tremendous reduction in active asthma and the need for medication. The placebo group, on the other hand, had virtually no change, displayed the same degree of active asthma, and therefore, still required the same degree of medical intervention.

Even more striking in this beautifully designed study is the data that continued to be gathered for the next seven years after treatment with the drops was finished (meaning that data was collected for ten years from the baseline, the start, of the study). Look at the SLIT (allergy drops) group. Ten years later, the majority of the group was asthma-free (the graph is mostly light gray)! However, ten years later, the control group is pretty much the same as when the study began—the graph is mostly dark gray, indicating that the children, now young adults, were still suffering from asthma to the same degree as they did when the study began.

This landmark study shows that we not only have the power to control allergic asthma by means of treatment with allergy drops, but that it can actually be reversed in the long term. Results like these affirm the promise of a new day for allergy and asthma sufferers.

Prevention Phase

It is exciting to think that in the future we will identify those children at risk for asthma and have the ability to intervene at a young age with sublingual allergy immunotherapy to prevent the asthma from developing, just like we developed vaccines for measles, mumps, and rubella. Well, the future is now! New research is showing how we can predict who will get asthma and how we can prevent it. But to prevent a problem, we must first realize a problem exists.

The Pediatric Asthma Crisis

According to an article that ran in *Time* on December 20, 2004, there are 6 million youngsters who suffer from asthma in the United States.[7] Asthma Action America—an organization of twenty-one health groups tracking asthma in this country—reported that 54 percent of asthmatic American children had had a severe attack in the past year and that 27 percent had had at least one attack that was so bad that they feared they were going to die. The report also stated that 71 percent of the youngsters and their parents didn't realize the severity of the problem. This incongruity was attributed to people's unawareness that environmental allergens such as dust mites or irritants from passive smoke exposure can trigger asthma, as well as their lack of knowledge about the differences between (and proper use of) rescue inhalers and preventive inhalers.

Up until now the greatest fear for a patient was "If my child has an episode of wheezing will he or she develop asthma?" The difficult part for pediatricians was that they couldn't answer that question. But this is changing. Dr. Fernando Martinez's important work in the Tucson Asthma Study has shown findings that are relevant for any young infant who wheezes. Parents of babies who wheeze are very concerned that their children will have asthma, which they know is a lifelong condition. Dr. Martinez and his group showed that the best predictor of whether an infant's wheeze will develop into asthma is the total IgE level in the first year of life.[8]

As you'll recall from earlier chapters, the total IgE represents the overall measure of allergy antibody in your blood, which is usually elevated in allergic people. In Martinez's study, the infants who had episodes of wheezing and who *also* had elevated total IgE were the most likely to develop persistent wheezing (asthma) as they got older. This clearly showed that the elevated allergy antibody put these infants at a greater risk for becoming asthmatic. But as we'll see, the risk of asthma also depends on environmental factors, and what the child is exposed to early in life has a great impact on what happens to him later.

Recent research is also showing that in children whose genetic predisposition (high IgE and TH2 predominance) makes them more likely to develop allergies and asthma, environmental exposure plays a significant role in determining whether they develop allergies and just what allergies they might be. For example, when given skin tests, many children with asthma test positive to dust mites, cockroaches, cat dander, and molds.[9,10] The sensitivity to these specific allergens increases the risk of asthma morbidity; these patient's allergies will exacerbate their asthma. An allergy-prone child who is exposed to cockroaches in his apartment building, lives with a cat, or sleeps with a mound of dust-mite-filled stuffed animals each night may be more likely to develop persistent asthma as a result of that exposure. On the other hand, environmental intervention that minimizes his exposure to these influences may tip the scale in the other direction, lessening the frequency and severity of his asthma flare-ups. There is documentation that shows an increase in severe asthma cases in Minneapolis during the fall season when mold spore counts were extremely high.[11] There is clear evidence of the connection between allergies and the development (and degree of severity) of asthma.

This is why it is so important to test patients for allergies, especially the younger ones and those who are at risk for asthma. If your doctor can identify the specific allergen to which your child is sensitive, she can teach you how to decrease your child's exposure. Even more important, there is evidence that you can reduce your child's symptoms by allergy immunotherapy.

Can We Predict Who Will Get Asthma?

A recent study by the collaborative group on the Prevention of Early Asthma in Kids, says there are indicators showing which young children are at higher risk for developing asthma.[12] The basis of the study was allergy and asthma questionnaire responses along with allergy skin test results. Among the 285 children enrolled, almost 61 percent (148) had a positive test to a food or environmental allergen. Additionally, the blood tests that measured the percentage of eosinophils and total IgE had the strongest correlation with allergy sensitization. And remember the study in chapter 1 from England and Sweden[13] researchers in that study found that children under five years of age who had high levels of three specific allergens—dust mites, dog, and cat allergens—were more likely to be persistent wheezers and hence become asthmatics.

The study group designed a table to categorize the children at highest risk for developing asthma:

The Asthma Predictive Index

1. The child must have a history of four or more wheezing episodes with at least one physical finding.
2. In addition, the child must have a history of four or more wheezing episodes with at least one physical finding confirmed by a physician.

The Modified Asthma Predictive Index: Major criteria
1. Parental history of asthma
2. Physician-diagnosed atopic dermatitis (eczema)
3. Allergic sensitization to at least one environmental allergen (dust mites, pollen, animals, etc.)

The Modified Asthma Predictive Index: Minor criteria
1. Allergic sensitization to milk, eggs, or peanuts
2. Wheezing unrelated to colds
3. Blood eosinophils greater than 4 percent in serum

I am not normally a big fan of using statistical tables for predicting or diagnosing conditions, because they tend to lump people into categories when each person is unique. However, in this instance, I do think that the Asthma Predictive Index serves the purpose of alerting parents whose children have early warning signs of allergies that they need to discuss with their pediatricians or general physicians whether their children are likely to develop asthma. The medical thinking now is that if allergy sensitization begins early in life, certain high-risk children initiate a perpetual allergic inflammatory response within the airways, and this can lead to the "allergic march" (remember, this is progression of allergies from the skin or intestinal tract in infants that can develop into rhinitis/sinusitis or asthma as the person reaches adulthood). For example, the study noted that boys from African American families showed 80 percent allergy sensitization four years after being followed in the group. This is significant because all the evidence indicates that childhood allergy sensitization means a higher likelihood of asthma later in life.

Can Sublingual Allergy Immunotherapy Also Prevent Asthma from Developing?

While it is important to identify children with allergies who are at risk for asthma, the real question is the one that follows from that: can we do anything to *prevent* the asthma once we identify those at risk of developing it? Though until recently the answer was no, new studies show that intervention with allergy drops can make a difference. An exciting new study in the *Journal of Allergy and Clinical Immunology* showed that children with seasonal hay fever (allergic rhinoconjunctivitis), who are at higher risk for developing asthma, can be shielded from this condition with the help of allergy drops (sublingual allergy immunotherapy).[14] The study took place in Italy, where children between the ages of five and fourteen who had hay fever as a response to grass pollen were followed over a three-year period. The experimental group received allergy drops to counter the effects of the grass pollen, and the control group received placebo (a sugar-water pill). The striking finding was that the group receiving the allergy drops was almost four times less likely to develop asthma. This study by Dr. Elio Novembre's group showed that the children receiving allergy drops had fewer hay fever symptoms during the grass pollen season, and because their allergies were being treated, they were less likely to develop asthma.

Your personalized Asthma Action Plan is the ideal first step in combating your symptoms and addressing the underlying cause. In the next chapter, we will explore the health conditions that often act like allergies and asthma, but are very different.

CHAPTER

8

Diseases That Masquerade as Asthma and Allergies . . . but Aren't

W e've already seen how frequently asthma escapes special notice and subsequent treatment because its symptoms are thought to be part of an infectious process. In these cases, a patient may be sent to many specialists before finally being referred to an allergist, although in this case the allergist will be the one who can help. Conversely, a patient with symptoms such as nasal or chest congestion, shortness of breath, and so forth that seem to scream allergy may go to an allergist and will learn that there is no evidence that the condition is allergic in origin. That's because some conditions "masquerade" as asthma and allergic rhinitis, and for these conditions allergy treatment, including immunotherapy, will be of no benefit.

In order to root out true allergy from other conditions that mimic allergies, it is essential to carefully take a patient history and perform a few key tests. As specialists in the field of allergy, we are also attuned to the signals that will raise the red flag, suggesting that something in the picture simply doesn't fit. For example, if a patient in his sixties without any prior history of allergy or asthma came to me with difficulty breathing, a red flag would go up for me. It is highly unusual that asthma would suddenly appear in someone of that age, so I would look to see if something else could explain these same symptoms.

If, after taking the complete history and doing an appropriate exam, I still suspect that allergic asthma does not fit the clinical picture of the patient that I am examining, there is one test that I find invaluable to confirming or ruling out that diagnosis: It is the pulmonary function test (PFT), or *spirometry*, that I mentioned above. This test measures the airflow through the bronchioles. The shape of the flow-volume curve is the basis used to establish whether you have the ability to breathe normally compared to what I like to call your "identical twin." The pulmonary function machine takes your personal information—height, age, and ethnicity—and calibrates (computes) the proper values that your ideal "identical twin" with normal breathing would produce.

As a general rule, our levels of IgE—the molecule that we know plays such a key role in allergies and asthma—naturally decrease by the time we are in our sixties, so it was unusual for allergies and asthma to suddenly develop at this age. If I were examining a patient in his sixties with symptoms of chronic coughing, shortness of breath, or wheezing, I would recommend a *pulmonary function test*. This is done with a simple machine that the patient blows

UPPER AND LOWER RESPIRATORY TRACT

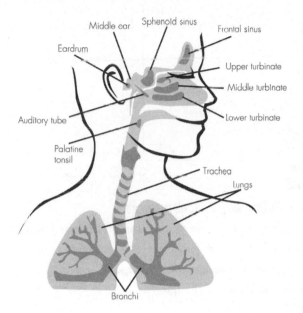

into. It records the person's lung capacity and the flow through the bronchioles. The test also provides special graphs that can indicate whether any compromised lung function is due to asthma or another lung problem.[1]

To understand the other conditions that may be masquerading as asthma it is helpful to survey the respiratory system. The diagram above shows you the entire respiratory tract. Doctors think of the respiratory system as having two parts, with the trachea, located in the center, being the dividing line. Any condition affecting the system *above* the trachea is considered an *upper respiratory tract* issue; everything *below* is described as belonging to the *lower respiratory tract.*

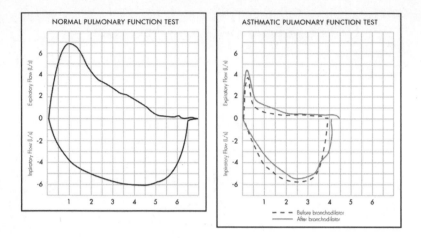

Normal Pulmonary Function Curve

Above left is an example of a normal pulmonary function test. The top half of the curve looks like a mountain, with a peak slanted slightly to the left and a straight slope "down the mountain"; it also looks like an isosceles triangle.

Pulmonary Function Curve in Asthma

By contrast, the diagram on the right is what you expect to see when you are looking at a patient with asthma. Do you see how the top of the triangle is very narrow in comparison to the normal picture next to it? The "collapsed" triangle in this picture indicates that less airflow is taking place, which indicates a blockage in the bronchioles. All of this is consistent with a diagnosis of asthma. A bronchodilator medication should reverse the blockage, and if this is found to occur it will also be consistent with the diagnosis of asthma, because asthma is a reversible condition.

The measurements taken by this test (called the *Forced Expiratory Volume* [FEV1], which is a fancy way of saying "the rate of air that you are able to blow out in one second"), are also important, because we want to see your rate reaching at least 80 percent of the one plotted for your "identical twin." If your reading is lower than that, you have an obstruction that may need to be treated.

The bottom curve (below zero on the *y* axis) is your *inspiratory loop*. Remember, asthma involves blockage when you breathe *out* (expiration), not when you breathe in (inspiration). The normal loop when you breathe in should look like a symmetrical semicircle; if this is shortened or irregular, then it indicates a problem that is higher up in the respiratory tract but is not asthma.

The pulmonary function test will also reveal other issues and may explain symptoms that look like asthma but aren't.

When Difficulty Breathing Is Not Asthma

In medicine we are trained to identify clusters of symptoms according to their most common diagnosis. Even the most astute medical diagnostician might be lulled into complacency if he saw a patient on a regular basis complaining of wheezing, shortness of breath, and coughing. That's why I find that it is so important to periodically review the initial diagnosis and the factors that led me to that diagnosis. (The medical truism that we must bear in mind is "All that wheezes isn't asthma.") There are other medical conditions that we will review below that can cause wheezing and will appear to look like allergic asthma—but aren't.

Heart Disease

If that same over-sixty patient we mentioned earlier comes to me with a possible history of long-standing hypertension, it may be that he has developed congestive heart failure, a condition in which the heart doesn't pump as efficiently as it should. In this case, fluid can back up into the lungs, which, during exertion, can cause shortness of breath (which presents like bronchial asthma), chronic cough, and wheezing. It is important to do a pulmonary function test to rule out bronchiole obstruction and, once that has been determined, to make sure that such a patient is referred to a cardiologist to get proper evaluation and medication to treat his heart condition.

This same condition can also occur in a younger patient if he or she has a severe heart valve deformity, or a more common condition called *IHSS (idiopathic hypertrophic cardiomyopathy)*. Listening to the patient's heart and discerning if there are any murmurs is critical to confirming that diagnosis. One of former President Clinton's first signs of heart disease was shortness of breath on his long daily walks—especially if there was an incline, like a hill. Dr. Daniel Berman's study in 1995 showed that in someone fifty years or older, shortness of breath may indicate heart disease.[2] It is important to be aware that patients with unexplained breathing problems have more than *twice* the risk of dying from cardiac (heart) causes as patients with chest pain. Why? Patients with chest pain are more likely to seek treatment. If you experience new shortness of breath, call your physician.

Gastroesophageal Reflux

I keep this diagnosis in the back of my mind when a patient isn't responding to regular asthma medications. Gastroesophageal, or gastric, reflux is now considered a well-known trigger for asthma,[3] yet it differs from typical asthma in that the condition has nothing to do directly with the lungs. The patient may have a hiatal hernia of the esophageal sphincter, an anatomical disorder that results in a reflux of stomach contents into the esophagus. That backup of acid causes irritation of the lining of the esophagus, which has nerves that interconnect with the nerves servicing the lungs (the *vagus nerves*) and can cause bronchospasm. Patients with reflux disease may also appear to be suffering from symptoms of asthma, usually in the form of chronic cough and throat clearing, and usually respond very well to acid-blocker medications. The newer medications like Nexium and Protonix seem to be especially effective. Of course, dietary changes such as giving up pepperoni pizza and soda are also important for these people. The tricky thing about diagnosing gastric reflux is that the patient doesn't necessarily have a history of heartburn. The condition may have existed as "silent reflux."

Anemia

If a patient's blood count is very low, it can lower the *perfusion* (blood flow) to the lungs, and this in turn can cause shortness of breath and even wheezing. The causes of anemia can be low iron due to loss of blood, vitamin deficiency (like B_{12} or folate deficiency), or a hereditary condition such as sickle-cell anemia.

The chief of my university medical department was a brilliant physician specializing in allergy admired for the breadth of his knowledge in all areas of medicine. He had an experience that perfectly underscores how easily even an expert can mistake anemia for allergy or asthma. In his case, the story began when he experienced occasional wheezing. It started in the spring when the pollen count was high, so he figured it was his rose fever (the spring equivalent of hay fever) allergy to grass that was triggering his symptoms. With the onset of wheezing he used an asthma inhaler, and each time, his wheezing would clear. However, a few months later, in the fall, he was getting more persistent wheezing and then, in addition, was experiencing some shortness of breath. He decided to treat himself with oral cortisone to get rid of this condition once and for all. But after a week of taking the cortisone, he still didn't feel much better. He finally relented and decided to see a colleague about his symptoms.

The doctor suggested that they do things the right way and do a full history and physical.

The doctor noticed on the exam that the professor had pale *conjunctiva* (eye membranes), and that his tongue was a glossy, shiny red—as opposed to its normal color of medium pink. The examining physician decided to do a blood draw, which confirmed his suspicion. The professor was very anemic. His blood count was 18, and the normal count for a man is 38. The professor's iron levels were normal, so there was no sign of blood loss, which could have explained an acute anemia. However, the shape of his blood cells was larger than usual. This indicated that he had a *macrocytic anemia*, which means he was deficient in either B_{12} or folate. Further tests revealed he had *pernicious anemia*, which is due to B_{12} deficiency. It's called "pernicious" because of its insidious onset, often with symptoms so subtle as to go unnoticed or be mistaken for something else. The happy ending to the story is that once the professor got his weekly B_{12} injections, his wheezing and other symptoms resolved.

Vocal Cord Paralysis

This sounds dreadful and lethal, but it's not. This condition can, however, easily fool even the most expert physicians into treating a patient for asthma, when in reality that's not the issue. The condition is more common in women than in men and also tends to occur more frequently in younger women (menstrual age to about twenty-five).[4] The actual cause can be anatomical. For example, several years after thyroid surgery, one of my patients presented with shortness of breath and wheezing, and her symptoms didn't respond to asthma medications. In addition, her pulmonary function test did not indicate a classic asthma pattern. She underwent a laryngoscopy, to see what may have been causing her condition. This is an exploratory procedure in which a tube is passed through the nose down the back of the throat so that the vocal cords can be seen. In my patient's case, the test revealed that her vocal cords weren't moving together properly and led us to a whole new diagnosis—vocal cord paralysis.

Alpha-1 Antitrypsin Deficiency

Alpha-1 antitrypsin deficiency (A1AD) can have an insidious onset: chronic coughing, difficulty breathing that worsens over time, recurrent respiratory infections that takes weeks to resolve. Many younger patients are diagnosed with asthma or episodes of bronchitis. However, a missed diagnosis in the early adulthood years can lead to *emphysema*, a devastating, irreversible lung disease. Emphysema is when the elastic recoil of the lungs is damaged and air gets trapped in the lungs and can't be exchanged for fresh air.

You may not have heard of A1AD, but because of my close association with doctors in the pulmonary department of the hospital where I trained, which was a special referral center for patients diagnosed with this condition, I saw many cases of it while training in my allergy fellowship. I was struck by how many years these patients had been labeled as asthmatics before an astute physician realized that they had been misdiagnosed and found the correct diagnosis.[5]

It is extremely important that any patient possibly having A1AD be tested for two reasons:

1. Left untreated, it can lead to irreversible emphysema at a young age (ages 30 to 50).
2. It can be effectively treated and controlled with a medication called Prolastin. It is the deficiency of this enzyme (alpha-1 antitrypsin) that causes erosion of the lining of the patient's lung tissue.

A simple blood test can show if a patient is deficient in this enzyme, and it can diagnose someone's genetic predisposition to develop the disease or to pass it along to their children. Elevated liver function test results provide other clues that the patient (even a child) may be at risk of developing this condition.

Sarcoidosis

Sarcoidosis is a lung condition that can be diagnosed in young adults. It can also present with symptoms that perfectly mimic asthma. It is more common among people of African American descent but can occur in all races. Besides chronic coughing or shortness of breath, other clues that can tip a patient or doctor off that this is not asthma involve the extrapulmonary findings.[6] Eye symptoms are commonly associated with sarcoidosis. These include *uveitis*, a painful condition in which exposure to light produces the feeling of being poked in the eye. Patients with sarcoidosis may also have rashes on the face or legs, which, to a dermatologist, would indicate the presence of this disease. Again, early diagnosis is the key, because this is a disease that flares up only intermittently but can produce blindness if not treated (with oral cortisone) in a timely manner. Sarcoidosis is classified as a restrictive lung disease (one in which the lungs don't fill up to maximal capacity) and is different from asthma, in which the lungs do fill up properly but the flow through the bronchioles is blocked. A pulmonary function test will easily differentiate these two conditions.

Cystic Fibrosis

Cystic fibrosis once meant an early death sentence for children, but now, thanks to early detection and aggressive treatment measures, patients can enjoy a normal life span.

The key medical indicator—outside of any related to the lung—that gives clue to this condition is "failure to thrive."[7] The term "failure to thrive" means the child does not grow in height or weight according to the standard pediatric growth-weight curves. The reason for this is that cystic fibrosis affects not only a child's lungs, but the pancreas as well. The pancreatic enzymes are blocked from being secreted, so food isn't digested and absorbed properly and chronic diarrhea results. In this disease, the patient's chloride channels in the lungs, pancreas, and skin are blocked. The definitive test to diagnose cystic fibrosis is a sweat test that measures the chloride ions in the skin after it has been stimulated with electric currents.

We've reviewed above the symptoms that look like asthma but are actually conditions that only mimic asthma—these are conditions that make you wheeze or experience other symptoms that are likely to make you and your doctor believe you are suffering from asthma. Conversely, the same sort of "masquerade" can occur in the upper respiratory tract so that you present with nasal symptoms that suggest allergy when that is not really the culprit.

Once again the lesson is that one can't always assume that a person with a chronic stuffy nose and a nasal drip has allergies. Let's review below some non-allergy-related conditions that can mimic allergic rhinitis.

When Chronic Stuffy Nose Is a Symptom of Something Else

Although symptoms may appear identical to the sorts of nasal conditions that we see in allergies, sometimes the problem is an overactive nervous tissue in the nose that causes it to swell up inside or to cause sneezing.[8] *Vasomotor rhinitis* is the common cause of sneezing when you get a whiff of that strong cologne that doesn't agree with your nostrils. It is also the cause of the sneezing that occurs when someone's nose gets congested going from hot to cold air, or vice versa. It's also the reason some people can't eat their delicious spicy meals without a tissue in hand. The special name for this variant is *gustatory rhinitis;* here, certain spices stimulate the sensory nervous tissue to trigger the release of neuropeptides in the mucus membranes of the nose, which results in a constant nasal drip.

Nasal Polyps

Nasal polyps occur when growths form on the mucus membranes within the nose. Besides nasal congestion, patients may have a diminished sense of smell (the medical term is *anosmia*) that makes food seem somewhat tasteless when they eat. By themselves, nasal polyps are not dangerous, but they do make nasal breathing a nightmare and, since the nasal secretions don't drain properly, can also predispose a patient to sinus infections. There is one thing that a doctor must be very careful about when examining a patient. If he finds a nasal polyp in one nostril, he needs to check for one on the other side. Nasal polyps are usually bilateral (occurring on both sides). If the polyp is only on one side and looks suspicious—not clear like a bubble—then it should be biopsied to rule out cancer. In my first year in practice, I diagnosed two locally invasive nasal cancers that appeared only on one side. Early detection saved these patients from extensive, disfiguring surgery.

Atrophic Rhinitis

Atrophic rhinitis is a condition that becomes more common as people age. The nasal tissue lining wears thin over the years, and as a result the person gets a runny nose when the temperature changes, when it gets very cold outdoors, or when exposed to indoor air-conditioning. Atrophic rhinitis is annoying, but not dangerous. The problem is that there isn't a good treatment for it, and saline nasal sprays are about the only solution that provides any relief.

Deviated Septum

A deviated septum can be another likely culprit behind chronic nasal congestion. If a patient comes to me complaining of a chronically runny or stuffy nose, I usually ask if they have had any recent trauma to the nose, perhaps because of a car accident, a skiing mishap, an accidental punch on the nose, and so forth. Boxers are well aware how much trauma to the nose can affect breathing. If, despite using prescription nasal sprays, you constantly feel you can't breathe through your nose, then it might be time to see an otolaryngologist (an ear, nose, and throat doctor) to have the deviated septum corrected.

It's important to remember that if you are not getting better with current treatment that is targeting your allergies or asthma, *tell your doctor,* because he or she may need to rethink the diagnosis. An old medical adage says that the third doctor you see for a problem is the best one. Why? By the time you see the third doctor, your symptoms and diagnosis are usually more obvious.

CHAPTER

9

Chronic Sinus Disease and the New Research

D id you ever have a cold that just hung on and on without getting better, even after five or more days had gone by? If you did, your doctor probably diagnosed you with an acute sinus infection and gave you antibiotics. Did the problem reoccur a few months later? How many times did you take antibiotics for cold or sinus problems in the last year? There is no set "right" number, but if you have taken three or more courses of antibiotics for this problem each year for the past several years, you may have a chronic sinus condition.

Acute sinusitis can occur after you have caught a cold. If it is viral in origin it will not require antibiotics. However, if the symptoms include headaches that are present when you wake up or head pain that comes when you bend over to pick something up, or if you experience pain when your forehead or cheek is touched, an ache in the upper teeth or jaw, and swelling around the eyes, then you may have a bacterial infection for which antibiotics are an appropriate treatment.

Chronic sinus disease, however, is a whole different ball game. Statistics show that 18 million cases of chronic sinusitis are treated annually in the United States, with at least 30 million courses of antibiotics prescribed, and that patients with chronic sinusitis scored worse on quality-of-life surveys and reported more pain than those with heart or lung disease or back pain.[1] Ouch! Chronic sinusitis can develop after an acute sinus infection, so bacteria may be the culprits. However, the main difference between acute and chronic sinusitis is in the mucus. The mucus in chronic sinusitis has been found to contain eosinophils, the presence of which indicates allergic inflammation. This surprising fact indicates that most cases of chronic sinusitis are *not* caused by a bacterial infection, and since the cause of the problem is not bacterial, *repeated courses of antibiotics will not help.* If the patient's condition is to be improved, the inflammation needs to be tamed.

"What's the harm in taking antibiotics just in case?" you may ask. "They're safe, aren't they?" The answer is that it's not that simple. Taking an antibiotic when you don't have a bacterial infection and don't need it just kills off "good" bacteria the body relies upon in the digestive system, Furthermore, though it will kill weaker bacteria that are hanging about in the body, the more resistant strains may survive to multiply and be more difficult to treat with antibiotics later on if you do develop bacterial infection.

Dr. Larry Borish at the University of Virginia Medical School has come up with a new way of thinking about sinus disease. He calls it "the asthma of the nose."[2] It has become common medical knowledge that asthma shouldn't be treated with antibiotics. Asthma is now treated with bronchodilators and inhaled cortisone to reduce the inflammation caused by our old allergy nemesis, eosinophils. Sinus specialists call chronic sinus disease *chronic eosinophilic hypertrophy sinusitis*, a mouthful of a phrase that more or less means "sinusitis caused by repeated swelling of the nasal sinuses caused by inflammation-fighting agents." The word *hypertrophy* is the medical term for swollen tissue, and it is believed that the eosinophil responds to inflammation in the sinuses and then causes the tissue to swell.

What causes the inflammation? Researchers at the Mayo Clinic did an important study to try to answer this question. When surgeons operated on patients with chronic sinus disease and polyps, they removed and examined some of the tissue (which they had first colored with special stains) under the microscope and found eosinophils. They also cultured the tissue and found that in 80 percent of cases it was predominantly fungi, not bacteria, that grew from it! Since fungi (molds) may act as allergens and trigger the inflammatory process, these new findings suggest that this form of sinus disease may be *allergic* in nature.[3]

Allergic Rhinitis and Chronic Sinus Disease

Drs. Ivor Emanuel and Saurabh Shah reviewed two hundred consecutive patients whose chronic sinusitis didn't respond to medicine and who had had sinus surgery. Allergy testing indicated that 84 percent of these people had a positive allergy test. The main allergens were year-round allergens, such as dust mites.[4]

In another study, Dr. J. Krouse did a study to evaluate the quality of life of patients with chronic sinusitis. Forty-eight patients underwent computerized tomography (CT) scans of their sinuses, were tested for allergies, and also completed a survey about whether their sinusitis disabled them. The findings showed that the allergy testing was a better indicator of severity of symptoms than the CT scan. This emphasized the importance of evaluating allergic disease and suggested that treatment of allergies may be key to the best outcome.[5]

Anatomical Facts

Jane Brody's recent *New York Times* article, "When Trouble Hits Those Holes in Your Head," makes the point that the four pairs of sinuses that lie in front of the skull are spaces filled with air, but when they are blocked, the mucus that may be secreted can't flow, and inflammation occurs.[6] To understand sinusitis, it is important to know some facial anatomy. Below is a schematic diagram of the four sinuses:

SINUS ANATOMY

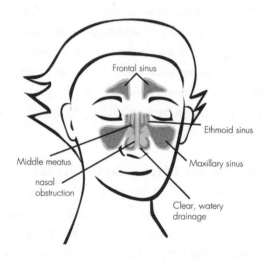

The diagram above shows the four paranasal sinuses, which exist in pairs. They are the *frontal sinuses,* which are located above the eye; the *ethmoid sinuses,* which surround the bridge of the nose; the *maxillary sinuses,* which lie below the facial cheek area; and the *sphenoid sinus,* which isn't seen here, but can be seen on a lateral view.

We don't yet understand the function of sinuses in the body other than that they are used in *phonation* (the production of speech), but their important locations, unusual anatomy, and varying shapes leave them vulnerable and easily compromised. The maxillary sinuses are the largest cavities of the group and are the most likely to become inflamed; they do so in 90 percent of sinusitis cases. The problem with these sinuses is that the mucus that accumulates at the bottom of the sinus must travel up against gravity through tiny canals called the *osteomeatal complex* to reach the ethmoid sinuses, into which they can eventually drain out. As you can see, the ethmoid sinuses are very tiny, narrow canals through which sinus fluids must make their way. They frequently become blocked, and their blockage is the cause of headaches and pain over the bridge of the nose. Though the sphenoid sinus is least likely to cause problems, it should not be overlooked. Just as can happen in a small pond in which fluids do not have the unrestricted movement they would have in a larger structure, the sinuses may be dammed up if the nasal tissue is swollen or the area is obstructed by polyps.

Nasal polyps are growths that can impede the flow of air and mucus in the sinuses. They are like little balloons that grow out of the patient's tissue, and they cause many problems, the most noticeable of which is difficulty breathing through the nose. They may also disable one's capacity to smell. Recurring infections, which are the most debilitating problem caused by nasal polyps, arise after the polyps become enlarged and block the sinuses from draining. ENT surgeons who remove polyps when they become large must warn the patient of the high likelihood that the polyps will re-form within five years.

During years of practice, I found that treating patients who develop nasal polyps could be difficult and frustrating, because the polyps almost always reoccurred after surgical or medical intervention. However, new hope for these patients is on the horizon because of the practice known as *aspirin desensitization*. It has been reported that 50 percent of patients with chronic sinusitis, nasal polyps, and asthma have sensitivity to aspirin and other nonsteroidal anti-inflammatory drugs, such as Ibuprofen. These chronic sinus patients with nasal polyps have an imbalance in the enzyme pathway that controls the production of chemicals involved in immune inflammation and produce an excessive amount of an enzyme called *leukotriene C4*. The leukotrienes are counterparts of the chemicals called *prostaglandins* that are involved in inflammation in muscles. Knowing this is important because it has been shown that if the leukotriene enzyme is blocked, which can be accomplished by aspirin desensitization, patients with nasal polyps, sinus disease, and aspirin sensitivity can have reduced symptoms, need fewer courses of antibiotics, require fewer surgeries, and regain the ability to smell and taste again.[7]

Aspirin desensitization is an oral technique whereby the patient is given an increasing dose of aspirin over several days until a therapeutic dose (usually 325 mg) is reached. When the patient is successfully desensitized, he is no longer sensitive to aspirin if he continues to take it regularly. The beauty of this is that aspirin at this dosage is already used for prevention of coronary artery disease and colon cancer. The additional benefit for the sinus patient is that his body will no longer produce excessive leukotriene enzymes, which cause eosinophils to enter his tissues and cause sinus inflammation and the development of nasal polyps.

Diagnosis

The best way to assess sinus disease is with a computerized tomography (CT) scan of the paranasal sinuses. The CT scan allows you to visualize each sinus. A normal sinus should appear black on the sinus CT, and areas that are cloudy or white indicate that the air spaces are blocked by inflamed tissue, fluid, or polyps. The red flags that suggest that you have a chronic problem and need a CT scan of the sinuses are:

1. Condition fails to improve after three months of medical therapy with antibiotics, decongestants, or nasal sprays.
2. Persistent pain in the face, headaches, and/or foul breath (halitosis).

The CT scan has been shown to have a good (85 percent) sensitivity at indicating sinus pathology. This knowledge is of great help in determining whether your treatment should make use of medications, surgery, or allergy immunotherapy.

Newer asthma medications called *leukotriene modifiers* may also help patients with chronic sinusitis, nasal polyps, and aspirin sensitivity. Singulair and Accolate are examples of such medications and have shown promise in terms of reducing symptoms. They work by restoring the proper balance between prostaglandin and leukotriene chemicals in the nasal tissue.

Treatments

My approach to helping the patient with sinus disease is to relieve nasal obstruction and treat the underlying allergens. I find that if my patients are to find relief, they must be able to do the following:

1. *Drain the sinuses:* This can be accomplished with the use of multiple nasal sprays. I usually start patients off with a combination of a decongestant spray, like Afrin, with a nasal steroid. The Afrin is critical to opening the patient's nasal and sinus tissue, for without this opening the nasal steroids won't penetrate deep enough to inhibit the inflammation and break up the mucus. I instruct my patients to use the Afrin for only three consecutive days and then

to stop so that they don't become "addicted" to this decongestant. The "addiction" is due to the rebound effect that can occur if any decongestant spray is used for weeks or months. The nasal steroids are used to decrease swelling and tissue inflammation; they are also what I like to call "mucus busters," because they break up thick mucus secretions and block the eosinophils from causing further inflammation. All of these sprays should be used under the proper supervision of your doctor.

2. *Increase fluid intake:* Patients should drink lots of liquids. Teas, thin soups, and bottles of water keep a person hydrated and help to thin mucus secretions and let them drain more easily.

3. *Wash the sinuses:* Saline nasal sprays help to moisten the nasal and sinus membranes, which loosens secretions and, according to some studies, helps protect people from getting viral infections. This cleansing can be done safely several times a day with no side effects. I strongly urge my patients with sinus problems that they do such nasal cleaning before, during, and after airplane flights. The dry, stale air of planes is murder on the sinuses.

4. *Humidify the air:* This also helps to loosen secretions as long as you keep the unit clean with a diluted solution of vinegar (one teaspoon vinegar for every cup of warm water) that prevents the growth of mold.

5. *Get steamed:* A hot shower's steam will open your sinuses and allow them to drain. Dr. Andrew Weil suggests using eucalyptus or thyme oil to assist with aromatherapy. (Add one drop of eucalyptus or thyme oil to a pot of water. Bring it to a boil on the stove, lower the heat to simmer; then stand over the pot with a towel placed over your head and breathe in the steam for about ten to fifteen minutes.)[8]

Can Allergy Drops Help?

To help answer this question, I turn to my mentor, Dr. David Morris. In conversations that I have had with Dr. Morris and during a lecture that he gave in 2002, he indicated that he believed chronic sinus conditions responded to treatment with oral antifungal medications like itraconazole (Sporanox) or fluconazole (Diflucan) to decrease the fungi in the nasal sinuses. He believes that reducing the fungus load in the sinuses will stop them from stimulating an immune response, as is the case with nail fungus infection. He believes this can be achieved safely by giving the oral antifungal medication twice a week. At this decreased frequency the treatment is beneficial without producing liver toxicity as a possible side effect. The second part of his approach is to use sublingual allergy immunotherapy (allergy drops) to specific fungal allergens like Alternaria, the most common mold, in order to build immune tolerance to these allergens.

The final word on the best treatment for chronic sinusitis has not yet been uttered, but as doctors move in on understanding the causes, the cures will follow. I need to add that I'm not a surgeon, but I have seen cases where extensive sinus disease and nasal polyps are alleviated with surgery—sometimes for good, sometimes temporarily. In the difficult cases, it can be helpful for the allergist and ENT physician to work closely together.

CHAPTER

10

Food Allergies

F ood allergies affect 11.4 million Americans, or 4 percent of the population. As the following table shows, these allergies are surprisingly prevalent compared to other common diseases.[1]

Disease	Number of People Affected
Cystic Fibrosis	30,000
Multiple Sclerosis	400,000
Juvenile (Type 1) Diabetes	1,000,000
Epilepsy	2,500,000
Heart Failure	5,000,000
Food Allergies	11,000,000

This chapter is very frustrating to write, because I have to state that up to now we have had no cure for food allergies. This means that *avoidance* is the only safe option for someone who is allergic to a specific food, and avoiding a particular food can be more difficult than most people realize. However, three new exciting treatments may greatly improve the quality of life for anyone with food allergies.

Before we discuss the new treatments, it's important to recognize what a food allergy reaction is, because it's not always obvious. Reactions caused by allergies to food run the gamut from rashes to diarrhea to death. The most common food allergies in children involve reactions to milk, eggs, soy products, peanuts, wheat, tree nuts, and fish. Adults are also allergic to these foods, and 6.5 million adults are allergic to shellfish and other fish.

In this chapter I will discuss some of the signs that indicate food allergies along with which foods are most commonly involved. Although most patients with allergies believe that food contributes to—or exacerbates—their problem, I tend to focus on food as a cause if the patients have the following clinical symptoms:

- skin rashes such as hives or eczema
- itching in the mouth
- vomiting or diarrhea during or shortly after a meal
- shortness of breath, wheezing, or swelling that develops during a meal or shortly afterward.

If a patient exhibits any of these symptoms, food allergy testing is in order. If hives and, sometimes, accompanying swelling (*angioedema*) occur acutely during or shortly after a meal, they may be due to a food allergy. The prime suspects in these cases are shellfish, nuts, and berries. Many people love to eat shrimp and lobster, but these high-protein foods are very allergenic to some people.

Nuts are another common, and dangerous, food allergen. Because they are high in protein they can cause explosive reactions in which hives develop and are quickly followed by swelling and breathing difficulty. I caution patients with nut allergies against eating out in restaurants, especially Asian restaurants, where nut oils are commonly used in dishes.

Eczema is the other common skin rash associated with allergies, especially children's allergies. Drs. Hugh Sampson and Allan Bock did some groundbreaking work that showed that food allergies were aggravating the rashes affecting infants and children with severe eczema. They used standard allergy testing (blood and skin tests) as well as a new technique called *double-blind placebo challenge* to show that when children with eczema ate certain foods, their eczema would flare up. Drs. Sampson and Bock gave these children capsules to swallow. Some contained various pulverized allergenic foods, while others contained a placebo filler. They administered these capsules without the patients or their doctors knowing which contained the suspect foods. The results showed that when these children ingested allergenic foods such as milk, eggs, wheat, soy, peanut, and fish, their eczema became worse. They followed up by demonstrating that when the children *avoided* the allergenic foods, the eczema lessened. This research turned many skeptical dermatologists into believers. Both doctors showed that when evaluating children with eczema, screening for food allergies is important.[2]

Among all the reactions to food that can occur, the respiratory responses are the most dangerous and frightening. They can present as shortness of breath, coughing, and wheezing. In most cases a patient undergoing such an allergic reaction will initially experience a rash or digestive problem (vomiting and diarrhea indicate that the body is trying to reject an allergen). However, instead of first showing such warning symptoms, some patients move directly into breathing difficulty, a situation that requires urgent medical attention.

Dr. Sampson has studied the data related to patients who have had acute allergic food reactions and found that response time has a real effect on the outcome.[3] In fact, delayed response can be fatal. Because of this, patients with known allergies to nuts and shellfish are commonly prescribed a device called an *EpiPen* that contains injectable adrenalin they can carry with them and administer to themselves if the need ever arises.

Epinephrine (adrenalin) is the medication of choice for treating a severe allergic reaction. Researchers have reviewed records from hospital emergency departments and found that only 16 percent of patients with severe allergies received epinephrine treatment in the emergency department; only 16 percent were given a prescription for epinephrine; and only 12 percent were referred to an allergist for follow-up care.

Whenever I see someone who has had a severe food allergy reaction, I take the time to show him or her how to use the EpiPen. I do this with a demonstrator EpiPen that does not contain a needle. I have the patients off take the gray cap that covers the tip of the instrument, and press the tip against their outer thigh until they hear a snap. I tell them that in a real situation that snap will indicate that the needle has gone in, and they will feel a pinch as it does. They are to count to ten, remove the EpiPen, and then call 911. One dose of epinephrine will work in 90 percent of cases, but a patient should be monitored at a medical facility for at least a few hours afterward. And the extra good news is that a study in 2005 by Dr. Estelle Simons (former president of the Academy of Allergy, Asthma, and Immunology) showed that sublingual epinephrine can work to reverse anaphylaxis[4]—"no more shots" is going mainstream.

Are Supplements Safe for Allergy Patients? (Or, My Aching Knees)

When discussing food allergies and their effects, it's important to understand that food is not just the meals you consume. Nutritional supplements are often made of food products, and foods can also be used in their processing.

Miguel was fifty years old when he came to see me because his lips and face were swelling up. He thought this must have been happening because of something he was eating, but he didn't know quite what. He loved Italian food and beef, chicken, and fish dishes; avoided shellfish altogether because he knew that eating crab would produce a similar type of swelling in him; and wondered whether Chinese food, or possibly a new ingredient in the tomato sauce he had been eating, was causing his problem.

We tested for food allergies and everything came back negative, except for the shellfish, which he already knew caused swelling. My best diagnosis at the time was that since many restaurants use the same pans to cook all the foods, maybe the Chinese food he was eating contained traces of juice from shellfish. I advised him to avoid Chinese food for a while and see what happened.

A few weeks later, he called me because the facial swelling had returned. "Doc," he said, "I swear, I didn't have any Chinese food. I've only eaten at home for the last few weeks." I asked Miguel to come in to be examined and gave him oral steroids to bring down the swelling. After I wrote the prescription, Miguel said, "You know, Doc, I forgot to tell you that I've had arthritis in my knees since walking the beat for twenty years on the police force. I've been taking these new supplements my wife says are good for arthritis: chondroitin sulfate and glucosamine." Since this was a new supplement at the time, I asked him if I could see the bottle, and there was our answer, written right on the label. *"Made from crab exoskeleton,"* the bottle said. The supplement was made of crushed crab shells! Miguel and I both smiled as we realized that this natural supplement was the cause of his problem. It was clear what he had to do. He never had another reoccurrence of the swelling.

Little Timmy's Story

One of my patients was a five-year-old boy with a known history of peanut allergy. His mother was as careful as she could be to ensure that he never had any peanuts. One day she took her son to an ice cream shop for a treat and ordered him an ice cream sundae without any nuts. Timmy enjoyed the first spoonful, but after the second he said, "Mommy, I don't feel good." His mother knew something was wrong. Her son was breaking out in hives all over his body and wheezing loudly. She checked the dish he had been eating from and saw Reese's Pieces, which contain peanuts, at the bottom of the sundae. She immediately put him in the car and raced to the nearest hospital. I met them there. Since it was known that he was having an allergic reaction, he received a dose of adrenalin, and his symptoms reversed.

These frightening episodes during severe allergic reactions are not that uncommon in children and adults with peanut allergy. Timmy's story is similar to incidents experienced by many young-sters who have life-threatening food allergies, but his story is impor-tant to share for other reasons as well.

Besides the medical problems, which were potentially fatal, Timmy had to overcome many other hardships related to his peanut allergy. At school he was ostracized as "the kid with peanut allergy," and he wasn't allowed to eat lunch in the school cafeteria, because the other children were allowed to bring in peanut butter sandwiches. Instead he had to eat alone in a study hall, with only a teacher for company. Timmy's early school years were lonely! Since it might have worsened his asthma, he couldn't participate in gym, either, and while the other kids were playing sports, he was back in study hall. He also had to take prednisone to control his asthma during severe flare-ups. Though the cortisone controlled his wheezing, he was very sensitive to it and his face would swell up whenever he had to use it, setting him even further apart from the others.

It tormented Timmy's mother to see her son suffering medically and socially. She would ask me, "Dr. Mitchell, will he make it?" I spent many moments reassuring her that, yes, we would get Timmy through these hard times to the better days that lay ahead.

Timmy was lucky to have a mother who loved him so much! She found as many ways as she could to make him feel special. When they were with me, she would announce that he was very helpful around the house, or tell me that he was a responsible and good student. Then I would say, "Keep working hard at school! By the time you're done, I'll need a good partner in my practice," and Timmy would smile and smile. He did have special qualities. He was a kind and sensitive boy. He was also very intelligent.

During Timmy's adolescence his asthma stabilized, and thanks to his continued vigilance regarding diet, he rarely had more episodes of food allergy. Meanwhile, he used his solitude well and continued to study hard and achieve excellent grades in school. Since he couldn't play outside in the cold weather months, he began lifting weights at home. Over time Timmy became strong and tall. By age fifteen, he was six feet in height. Lifting weights had given him power, and now he made the football and lacrosse teams! He was also an outstanding student and was made a presidential scholar and sent to Europe to represent America's youth.

Timmy had to overcome many obstacles to become the fine young man he is today. Fortunately, there now are laws that protect children with food allergies from discrimination. The Food Allergy Network is an organization that works tirelessly to ensure that children with food allergies are protected in schools and airplanes, and it also has safeguarded them because manufacturers have been pressured to disclose all the ingredients in food products.

Of course, children aren't the only ones who are susceptible to food allergies.

Sometimes a Patient's Reaction Is Not So Obvious; Or, The All-American Sandwich

Lacey was a thirty-five-year-old singer who came to me after her internist became concerned about her persistent asthma. Lacey felt her condition was limiting her ability to sing at peak level. When I listened to her history, I learned that her nasal allergy symptoms and asthma got worse in the spring and fall when the pollen counts were the highest. However, this didn't explain why she had asthma all year long, since pollen is not in the air all of the time. During the physical exam, I examined her lungs and heard wheezing sounds, which indicated a partial blockage of the airways. We took a blood sample to be analyzed for environmental allergies. I also decided to do tests for food allergies, because she had told me that she occasionally developed hives. I told her to continue with the asthma inhaler she had been using. On her follow-up visit two weeks later, we discussed all the tests that had come back positive. She was allergic to trees, grass, and ragweed pollen, which made sense given what we both knew about her history. However, some food allergy tests were also positive. When I told her that she was allergic to tomatoes, wheat, and peanuts, she started to laugh "I eat peanut butter and jelly sandwiches on wheat bread every day for lunch," she told me.

It was surprising that Lacey had never noticed any acute reactions after eating those daily sandwiches, but now she knew better than to eat them. She left my office, promising to keep away from the sandwiches and continue her medications. When she came back to see me a month later, Lacey was grinning from ear to ear. She told me that she was so much better that she didn't even need her asthma inhalers.

"I didn't tell you to stop your inhalers," I replied, with some trepidation. She had taken them for the first week, she told me, but then the change in diet had left her feeling so good that she didn't need the inhaler. I was skeptical, but when I checked her lungs, they were clear, with good, clear breath sounds. This was one of the few times that I have seen a particular food allergen play such a dramatic role in a patient's allergic asthma.

These two stories show the extent to which food allergies can affect people's life. Little Timmy, who is now big Timmy, underwent many allergic episodes, some of which were so daunting that he and his mother had to live in fear. The good news for Timmy and other patients with peanut allergy is that two new treatments provide a measure of security they did not have before.

Future Treatments

Since allergic reactions to peanuts have been known to be life-threatening, I am glad to say that three promising treatments for all food allergies—one based on a hi-tech monoclonal antibody, another on an ancient Chinese herbal formula, and the third being sublingual allergy immunotherapy—are currently under investigation and may be available to patients in the near future.

Anti-IgE

Anti-IgE is an important treatment in the testing phase that may offer hope for people with food allergies. Unfortunately, due to patent disputes, its marketability is in limbo. However, it does indicate that potentially effective treatments are in the pipeline, and there is hope for the future.

This treatment, which was discussed in the *New England Journal of Medicine* in March of 2003, was based on the biology of monoclonal antibodies.[5] These antibodies are made to bind to IgE (the allergy antibody) and block IgE from binding to cells that have IgE receptors. By blocking the IgE receptors, the allergic chemicals aren't released and, theoretically, no allergic reaction occurs.

Dr. Leung along with Dr. Sampson and others set up double-blind studies with two groups of peanut-allergic patients. The experimental groups received different doses of the anti-IgE compound (known as TNX-901), and the control group received placebo injections. The experimental group that received the highest doses of anti-IgE before being challenged with peanut flour didn't develop allergic symptoms until they had eaten the *eighth* peanut. This was incredibly exciting news, because normally if any of these patients had ingested even a small piece of a peanut, they could, and usually would, have developed a strong allergic reaction. Though the exact times are still to be determined, the treatment seems to protect people from dangerous reactions to peanut exposure for as long as five weeks. Dr. Sampson has also reported that volunteers who received anti-IgE in the study said they had developed a greater tolerance to other food allergies besides peanuts!

Unfortunately, this promising therapy cannot be offered to the public until two issues are resolved. The first is a scientific one and involves establishing the periods of time during which people have to remain in treatment. The other is a legal matter. Because three companies are fighting over the patent for this treatment, the phase three research, which must be completed before general public use can be considered, has been halted until the patent issue is resolved.

Chinese Herbal Formula

A second treatment that is being studied (at Mount Sinai's Jaffe Food Allergy Center) is a Chinese herbal formula. The formula, originally called *FAHF-1* (*food allergy herbal formula*), was shown to block peanut-induced anaphylaxis in mice. The researchers recently refined this formula and called it *FAHF-2*. What was astonishing is that when mice that were bred to be peanut-allergic and develop anaphylaxis from peanuts were first treated with FAHF-2, they didn't develop any signs of anaphylaxis. The protection lasted up to five weeks.[6]

These results are of great interest, but of course the real excitement will begin when the treatment gets approval for testing on humans. Since the number of cases of food-induced anaphylaxis has doubled between 1997 to 2002 and now affects three million Americans, and peanut anaphylaxis accounts for 66 percent of that, we hope that this therapy will be on the fast track for clinical trials.

Sublingual Allergy Immunotherapy

The final therapy for food allergies is near and dear to my heart: sublingual allergy immunotherapy. Researchers from Spain did a daring yet beautiful study trying to help patients with a history of hazelnut food allergy. Hazelnut is very common in packaged foods, especially in candy bars, and it can be very dangerous. The study looked at twenty-three patients with hazelnut allergy confirmed by allergy testing. One group received sublingual allergy immunotherapy, and the other received placebo drops. The treatment was done in a rush protocol over four days in the hospital, and the study participants continued a home program for an additional eight to twelve weeks. The exciting findings were that nearly 50 percent of the treated group were able to tolerate 20 milligrams of hazelnut (the highest dose), whereas only 9 percent of the control group could handle that dose. This study holds promise for patients with severe nut allergy.[7]

Another type of food reaction that is more likely to occur in patients who have environmental allergies is called the *oral food allergy syndrome*. When these patients bite into an apple and start to chew it, they begin to experience itching in the mouth. They don't usually get a rash, and the effect doesn't usually progress to a more serious reaction, but it is uncomfortable. The oral itching is not due to pesticides on the apples, as many patients believe. It is due to the cross-reacting allergen that exists in patients who have sensitivity to birch tree pollen. Not all patients who test positively to birch tree pollen have the oral allergy syndrome; but in most cases the patient who responds to the apple with oral itching has the birch tree pollen allergy. Other common fruits that cross-react with the birch tree pollen are pears, kiwis, apricots, cherries, and plums, as well as carrots, celery, soybeans, and hazelnuts.[8] If you have any of these known food allergies, pay attention to what happens to you in the spring. If you notice that you then start sneezing or have watery eyes, it all makes sense when you know about oral allergy syndrome. You're not crazy!

Other pollen cross-reactions include ragweed with bananas, watermelon, cantaloupe, honeydew, zucchini, and cucumber. Sometimes a person will notice that they can't eat a particular food during the ragweed season, which goes from mid-August until mid-October, but that they can have it at other times. Grass pollen, which occurs in May and June, cross-reacts with peaches, potatoes, and tomatoes. A rare cross-reaction that I have never actually seen in my practice occurs between dust mites and shrimp.

Foods that cause oral itching when eaten raw can sometimes be eaten without causing those symptoms if cooked. For example, a patient with the oral allergy syndrome to apples can usually eat apple pie, because cooking breaks down the protein that causes the allergic reaction. It is important to note that this only applies to fruits, not to nuts or shrimp.

When Allergies Look Like Something Else:
The Vegetarian Surgeon

Strangely enough, having an allergic reaction to a food may not be a food allergy per se. This is why it is important to partner with a physician or allergist who can eliminate the nonallergens and focus in on the true cause of your reaction.

Several years ago, I had a patient who was an eye surgeon. He came to me because over the last few years he had begun following a strictly vegetarian diet and had recently noticed that he was having reactions to many foods he had previously eaten without any problems. He noticed that cherries, plums, carrots, and celery all made his mouth itch. Then he noticed that eating bananas with cereal made him itch. Strangely enough, he also felt his work was being affected. When he was working in the operating room, his eyes would begin to bother him until, toward the end of the surgery, they felt itchy and swollen. When I heard about the combination of his food allergies, especially regarding bananas, with his occupation as a surgeon, I diagnosed latex allergy, since it is commonly associated with food allergies to bananas, avocados, chestnuts, kiwis, and papaya.

Latex allergy has become a serious health hazard within the medical profession. It manifests when a person becomes allergic to the natural rubber latex found in rubber gloves and other rubber products. It is an important, increasingly common, and potentially deadly allergy. It is easily overlooked, and sometimes food allergies are the initial presentation. The doctor was relieved when I made this diagnosis. Now that he understood the problem, he and the other operating room staff began using non-latex gloves so they would have a latex-free environment when they operated. My patient's symptoms abated. Personally and professionally, he felt much better.

A Food That's Not a Food: The Tale of the Allergist's Wife

Vitamins are generally safe and healthy, but if you have food allergies it's important to know all the ingredients your vitamins contain—and sometimes that doesn't easily solve the issue. Being vigilant is the only thing that is going to work for you. Here's a story from another allergist, who dreads seeing certain vitamins because of his firsthand experience.

The allergist was having dinner with his wife in a coffee shop one day. She was eating some split pea soup when she began to experience an intense itching in the throat. Since she had a history of asthma and was beginning to notice some tightness in her chest as well, she used her Albuterol inhaler. But in spite of the medicine, the feeling of heaviness kept intensifying. She asked her husband if they could step outside for some fresh air. After a few minutes on the sidewalk, she fell to the ground and had to be rushed to the hospital, where, most fortunately, she was revived with oxygen and adrenaline.

It had been a terrifying incident. She had gone into allergic shock, but what was the cause? Her husband, who is a brilliant allergist, did the testing and found to his astonishment that she was allergic to carrots! It seemed that the carrots in the soup had triggered the reaction. It was a close call, but it wasn't the end of the story. The allergist's wife was careful not to eat carrots again, but when she felt a respiratory infection coming on a few weeks later, she decided to take some preventive measures to fend off a flare-up of the asthma. She would use her inhaler, of course, but besides that, she decided to buy some vitamins. She figured that a multivitamin with extra vitamin C might help, and as soon as she bought them, she popped one into her mouth. Soon thereafter, she was down again, in the same life-threatening state she'd experienced when she reacted to the carrots, only this one came on faster. She had to be rushed to the emergency room again. When her husband got to her side, he asked, "You didn't eat anything with carrots, did you?" "Of course not," she replied. "I didn't have anything except a vitamin for my cold." Her husband, the allergist-detective, rummaged for the bottle in her bag. The multivitamin tablets contained beta-carotene, the main vitamin in carrots. This must have triggered the reaction. As she would say later, "Who could have known?"

Clearly, allergic reactions can result after eating certain foods or taking certain vitamins and supplements. They can also stem from certain additives that are put in food for flavoring or as preservatives to keep the food fresher longer. For example, many people have experienced aches and pains after eating Chinese food containing MSG (monosodium glutamate), a flavor enhancer that has caused many such allergic reactions.

The Sulfite Story;
Or, Take Me Out to the Ball Game, but Hold the Sauerkraut

Stephanie enjoyed going to baseball games with her husband. It was much better than staying home alone. He was a big Mets fan, and over the years she had become one, too. She was in her early fifties and in reasonably good health, except for mild, intermittent asthma. The asthma usually presented with chronic coughing that would lead to wheezing and shortness of breath during cold weather or when she had developed an infection. However, on some of those beautiful summer nights after the ball game, she began to notice that she was getting her cough back and having difficulty breathing. The shortness of breath would develop later on in the evening, and she would have to use her asthma pump. She couldn't figure out why this was happening. Was she getting too excited at the games? Or could it be something she was eating there?

She decided to take action and came to the allergy clinic in New York City where I was training at the time. In the small cubicle that served as my office she informed me that the asthma attacks seemed to coincide with going to Mets games. When I joked that maybe it had to do with their recent losing streak, Stephanie grimaced like a true fan, before breaking out into a grin. "I don't mind the games," she said, "but to tell you the truth, I really go there for the hot dogs and a beer." I asked her if she ate hot dogs at other times. "Not really," she replied, "I eat them at the games because they smell so good and taste delicious with sauerkraut on top—but they are so fattening!"

I now suspected the hot dog was our culprit. Hot dogs are usually made from pork, which is a common allergen, however, since Stephanie's response to the food was always delayed, I suspected the preservatives. The hot dog has

continues

---

nitrates, but they don't normally cause allergic or asthmatic reactions. Sauer-kraut, however, is loaded with *metabisulfites.* Metabisulfites or sulfites are com-monly used to preserve food's color and keep it from spoiling. They were once used in open salad bars until they caused so many problems that adding them was banned. Other common foods that have high sulfite counts are dried fruits (except for raisins and prunes), maraschino cherries, shrimp, vinegar, wine, beer, and sauerkraut, which happens to have one of the highest sulfite levels of all.

I was pretty sure of my diagnosis, but because Stephanie loved her sauer-kraut, we arranged to do a metabisulfite challenge test to be sure. This is a pro-tocol during which the patient is given small increments of sulfite in a capsule, alternating with a placebo. If at a certain dose the symptoms develop, then we have a positive diagnosis. In Stephanie's case it took only two capsules before she started to cough and wheeze. I gave her a bronchodilator treatment to reverse the symptoms, but we had made the diagnosis. Since Stephanie had already tested negative for pork, we now knew which food was causing her problem. Later that summer she was back at the ball games, but this time she told the hot dog vendor, "Hold the sauerkraut."

There *Is* Good News for Food Allergy Sufferers

While this chapter has been full of examples of how you must remain vigilant and how there are many hidden places where food allergies lie, there is good news to report. You are not alone. There are two groups fighting in your corner, the Food Allergy Initiative (FAI, www.FoodAllergyInitiative.org) and the Food Allergy Network (FAN, www.FoodAllergy.org), an organization started by a group of mothers whose children suffered from food allergies. They have made the world safer for any person with a food allergy. These groups fund research to find cures for food allergies. The network has a newsletter that alerts its members when manufacturers misplace or mislabel ingredients in a food product. For example, if a batch of chocolate candy bars from a company gets accidentally mixed in with peanuts, which could be deadly for a peanut-allergic person, the company sends this information to the Food Allergy Network, which gets the information out to its members and to the public.

I admire the tenacity of these organizations. They enable people with food allergies to feel more secure in what they eat. As an allergist, I find these groups to be a valuable resource for myself and my patients. The take-home message from the Food Allergy Network is *read the labels if you have food allergies!*

CHAPTER 11

Your Better Breathing Program

I was fascinated when I read Dr. Andrew Weil's *Spontaneous Healing* and he described watching Dr. Robert Fulford, an osteopathic physician in his eighties healing patients through manipulation, breath work, and exercises. In fact, Dr. Fulford's unforgettable quote was, "The key to being healthy resides in the breath."[1,2] It sounds so easy, but we all know that a major opponent to better breathing is stress.

The Hidden Dangers of Stress, and How You Can Learn to Breathe Easy

Think back to the periods in your life when you were experiencing stress at great levels, and how your body felt at the end of the day. Most likely, you felt run-down and utterly beaten as you retired to bed, and if the stress stretched over an extended period of time, you can probably remember becoming or feeling quite ill. At the time, you most likely cursed fate for bringing you such misfortune. "Great!" you probably said, "Just what I need."

You may find it surprising that rather than illness occurring simultaneously with your period of high stress because of a stroke of bad luck, the two were quite possibly correlated. In recent years, studies have revealed that your stress level is indelibly linked to your body's ability to resist attack from illness. Perhaps more important to you is the link between stress levels and the onset of asthma attacks. Yes, there is one—and a very strong one, in fact.

In this chapter you will come to understand exactly how stress can affect your asthma. You will also be introduced to a surprisingly simple and enjoyable two-step relaxation regimen that you can easily incorporate into your daily life. I have used the program with great success with my patients, who as a result have developed greater tolerance for stress and, simultaneously, greater resistance to the uninvited asthma attacks that stress can produce.

The Stress Connection

Stress plays an important role in affecting our health; the research is clear on that. It seems no body organ is spared the effects of stress, but since each one of us has particular susceptibilities, the effects vary from person to person. Stress does its harm according to those weaknesses. In the mid-1990s I was very interested in the affect stress had on the body, and I attended several workshops held by medical professionals doing exceptional research on how stress could cause illnesses, as well as natural ways of relieving those stresses.

The first workshop took me to California, where Dr. Dean Ornish had developed his Program for Reversing Heart Disease. In his research Dr. Ornish had shown that in patients with coronary artery disease (blocked vessels to the heart), pain could be lessened and arterial blockages reversed when his patients ate a vegetarian diet, practiced yoga, and had group support.[3] At first, conventional cardiologists called his ideas ludicrous. However, they ceased their nay saying after reviewing the high-technology PET (positron-emission tomography) scans that proved that heart disease reversal had actually occurred among the participants in his investigations. When I arrived in Berkley, California, to attend Dr. Ornish's meetings, I expected to be handed some secret formula that had helped these patients. Instead, I learned of the techniques and lifestyle changes that had helped these patients handle the stress that literally had been killing them.

My next stop in understanding the powerful relationship between stress and illness led me to the Stress Reduction Program led by Dr. Jon Kabat-Zinn. While working out of the University of Massachusetts, Dr. Kabat-Zinn took on the unique challenge of aiding people who suffered from chronic pain from various injuries or cancer through a program that used mindfulness meditation. This ancient Buddhist practice that had existed for twenty-five hundred years was being employed in mainstream medicine for the first time. In his stress reduction clinics Dr. Kabat-Zinn taught mindfulness meditation to his patients and was able to show that the daily practice of meditation and yoga demonstrably improved their quality of life.[4]

I returned to Massachusetts to learn more at the Harvard-affiliated Deaconess Hospital, where Dr. Herbert Benson had been working for several decades on lowering patients' blood pressure using a form of meditation he termed "The Relaxation Response." Dr. Benson had gone to Tibet to study the Buddhist monks there and had found that once they achieved a deep form of relaxation, they could do amazing things with their bodies. He then brought some of these monks back to his lab at Harvard, hooked them up to electrodes, and measured their body temperatures and blood pressures during various states of consciousness. He found that the monks experienced amazing physical effects produced by deep meditative states, which lowered their blood pressure and heart rates. Dr. Benson has spent the last twenty years adapting these findings and using them in his clinics. He teaches his relaxation response to patients so that they can use it to lessen the stress in their lives and reverse overly high blood pressure and other illnesses brought on by stress.[5]

Witnessing these doctors' work made a deep impression on me. I was fortunate to have had the opportunity to see firsthand that the body was capable of breaking down under stress, and to learn how stress and its injurious effects could be modified. I then started to run my own wellness programs, where I brought in experienced instructors to teach my patients yoga and meditation—I even taught some classes myself. Not surprisingly, the majority of people who signed up were patients in my practice with allergies and asthma.

It was exciting to see a different side of my patients—doing the exercises and feeling they didn't need their medications as much. One man in particular, Peter, was a high school teacher with a calm exterior but an explosive temper. He told me stories of how when the teenagers in class got him angry, he would have to reach for his inhaler and take a few puffs as he felt his chest tightening up. He participated in our wellness program and found it enjoyable. But the big payoff came several months later: at school, he got into an altercation with a student who was disruptive. He and the student were called to the principal's office to discuss the matter. Peter could feel his chest tightening, and as he was about to reach for his inhaler he remembered the breathing techniques we taught him. He found an empty classroom and for a few minutes quietly did his breathing exercises. After about ten minutes, he felt his chest was more open and he didn't need his inhaler. He was also able to handle the meeting with his principal in a more composed manner.

Dr. John Sarno, a doctor who practices in New York City, has affected my practice greatly. When I was a medical resident, I attended his seminars on treating back pain. At the time, I was suffering from severe back pain: I had tried all types of physical therapy with limited improvement, but it wasn't until I read Dr. Sarno's book and attended his seminars that I began to understand the psychological impact that emotions have on pain and disease.[6] Dr. Sarno also described interesting parallels with other conditions, similar to back pain, that were noted to have an emotional component: ulcers, colitis, headaches, allergies, and asthma. And although some conventional doctors thought Dr. Sarno's work was quackery, his following of patients and their remarkable stories spoke for themselves. The core of Dr. Sarno's work is to help the patient understand that the pain or illness is meant to be a distraction from something the patient's unconscious doesn't want to be revealed; once this "something" is brought to light through education or psychotherapy, the pain will go away.

Drs. Ornish, Kabat-Zinn, Benson, and Sarno had unknowingly become pioneers in the new field of *psychoneuroimmunology*.

Psychoneuroimmunology (PNI)

Psychoneuroimmunology encompasses the fields of behavioral medicine (*psych*), and the nervous (*neuro*) and immune system. For decades, doctors saw these systems as separate and distinct. Western medicine was built on the idea that the mind and body were separate, and that the body was to be treated like an automobile—if one part breaks down, just fix that part.

Today we know better. The field of mind-body medicine started to emerge when researchers began finding scientific proof that the brain and the rest of the body were intimately working together. Dr. Candace Pert and fellow researchers at the National Institutes of Health showed that small proteins used as messengers in the brain, neuropeptides, were also found in the digestive system.[7] What were these neuropeptides doing in both places? Obviously, the brain has something to say about what goes on in the gut and vice versa.

A shocking finding made over ten years ago made by Dr. David Felton at the University of Rochester Medical School was the finding of nervous tissue in the spleen on a sample of a pathology slide.[8] The reason this was so fascinating is that the spleen has always been associated as an immune organ, and to find nerve tissue connected inside meant that the nervous system was clearly wired to the immune system and communicating!

BRAIN SCANS FIND SPOT THAT LINKS STRESS AND ASTHMA

This was the headline in the science section of the *New York Times* on September 6, 2005. The article was a preview of the paper being published the following week in the prestigious *Proceedings of the National Academy of Sciences*. Using brain-scanning techniques, researchers located a specific part of the brain that causes people with asthma to wheeze when under emotional stress.

Asthma sufferers often note that anxiety and emotional turmoil make the symptoms of an attack much worse. In the above study, Dr. Melissa Rosenkranz and her group from the University of Wisconsin showed that when people with asthma are exposed to their allergen, it activates certain centers in the brain that are intimately involved in emotions.[9]

The researchers exposed six volunteers with mild allergic asthma to two different substances: first, methacholine, which causes bronchial constriction, and second, a specific allergen that would cause inflammation. At one hour, during the constrictive phase, a functional MRI was done, and at four hours another MRI was done, during the inflammation stage. The functional MRI took active pictures of the brain's activity. During the scans the volunteers were asked to read words on a screen. The words ranged from emotionally neutral, like "curtains," to negative emotional words, such as "lonesome," and some words were specifically associated with asthma; for instance, "wheeze," "cough," or "suffocate."

Talk to Your Brain . . . It's Not Insane!

The interesting finding was that the presentation of words specifically associated with asthma attacks caused an increased activity in the inflammatory phase in a part of the brain called the *anterior cingulated cortex* (ACC), which governs emotions. This did not occur when subjects read neutral or negative words.

Researchers at Stanford University have taken these findings a step further by teaching volunteers MRI-assisted brain exercises to improve a person's control over a specific brain region.[10]

Extra Stress from an Extraterrestrial: Can Movies Trigger Asthma?

The link between psychological stress and asthma was cleverly revealed in a study done by Dr. Bruce Miller and his associates at the University of Buffalo. He studied twenty-four children with moderate to severe asthma who were asked to view the movie *E.T. the Extra-Terrestrial*—a film well known as an emotional roller coaster. The researchers monitored the children's heart rate, respiratory rate, and oxygen saturation—all parameters assessing their anxiety and asthma. The children were shown four scenes: (1) the opening credits (neutral); (2) E.T. death scene (sadness, hopelessness); (3) E.T. revival scene (happiness); and (4) E.T. departure (happiness and sadness). Dr. Miller found that the children had greater difficulty breathing when there were scenes of sadness and hopelessness, as compared to the happy or neutral scenes.[11]

Another study by Dr. Miller and Beatrice Wood, PhD, again showed *E.T.* to a group of children with asthma, but this time researchers videotaped each child in an emotionally challenging family task. They found that children with asthma who blamed themselves for a family disturbance were at increased risk for an asthma attack.[12]

The Holmes-Rahe Stress Index

In 1967 Drs. Thomas Holmes and Richard Rahe, psychiatrists at the University of Washington Medical School, had studied the role of stress on illness and devised a scale (the Holmes-Rahe Stress Index) to assess the likelihood that a person would develop an illness due to her stress level. Heading the list is death of a spouse. The doctors found that widows and widowers were ten times more likely to die after the death of a husband or wife. Also, divorced people experience illness twelve times more frequently than those who were married. The doctors noted that change—whether good or bad—causes stress, ultimately making us more susceptible to disease.[13]

Helen's Story: Love and Marriage

The stress in people's lives can have profound effects on their health. The mind and the body don't always differentiate between positive and negative stress. The following story about my patient Helen emphasizes this point. Helen's general doctor referred her to me because for six months she had experienced swelling all over her body (the medical term is *angioedema*) as well as hives (rashes that look like giant mosquito bites). I took a thorough history to identify any possible trigger for her skin reactions. However, there was no clear-cut food, drug, or vitamin supplement that could explain her condition. I did extensive allergy testing on Helen to see if there was an allergic cause to her symptoms. All of her food and environmental allergy tests were negative. I also checked her liver and kidney tests to make sure there were no internal malfunctions. All tests were normal. Helen was frustrated. The only way she could control the symptoms was by taking oral cortisone, which she knew had side effects if taken for long periods of time.

By her third visit, Helen and I felt more comfortable in our doctor-patient relationship, and I asked her if she felt under more stress than usual. She was a woman who appeared calm on the outside and spoke softly without much emotion. At first she denied any major stresses in her life, and I began to outline a plan with medications to try to better control her swelling. But just before we concluded the visit, she said, "I don't know if this makes a difference, but I'm getting remarried in two months. He and I have been dating for several years. The only thing is that he has three teenage boys and I have three teenage girls—a real Brady Bunch, except we don't have Alice the maid." We both laughed at that. She also added, "I don't know if this matters, but I was doing very well at work in this real estate office. They promoted me to manager and whereas before I just made my own sales, now I'm responsible for forty sales people."

I explained to Helen that this was all very significant information. The allergy immune system and the nervous system closely communicated. In the past her condition was called *angioneurotic edema;* the *neurotic* part was because doctors treating these patients noticed an association between these swelling attacks and emotional stress, for example, an argument with a spouse or a fight at work. The term *neurotic* was later removed from this diagnosis because it was discovered that these attacks can be due to a deficiency— inherited or acquired (a protein component of the immune system)—and doctors wanted to remove the stigma of a psychological term in the diagnosis. Nevertheless, many doctors have forgotten the importance of stress in triggering these attacks.

In Helen's case I came up with a medication program to control the hives and swelling until her wedding. I gently told her I thought the condition would improve once she acclimated to her new home and job situation. She gave me a look that said, "I'd like to believe you." I did recommend she learn some of the breathing techniques I was teaching other patients in our evening classes, saying that they might help ease her stress.

I spoke to Helen three months after her wedding. Her hives and swelling were gone. Life was more hectic than before, but she said, "I think the anxiety and anticipation were the worst part; now I know what I'm in for and can handle it better." The psychological component and the role of stress and emotions in any illness is something that should not be overlooked. Helen called me on rare occasions when her swelling reoccurred—most likely related to stress. On these occasions (thankfully, rarer), we used the Holmes-Rahe Stress Index to assess the severity of her stress level and to determine if she was at risk for disease as a result of it.

The Holmes-Rahe Stress Index scale sets up a point system to assess who is at greatest risk for illness related to the stress in their lives. The higher your score, the more likely you can develop a stress-related illness. If you have several events in a short period of time, you have an even greater likelihood of developing an illness. In Helen's case we saw that getting married, which is usually considered a joyous event, is actually quite stressful and carries a 50-point score on the stress index; in addition, she took an extra responsibility at work, which carried with it an extra 36 points. So in a short period of time, she had accumulated 86 points on the stress index scale. She was a likely candidate for a stress-induced illness.

Holmes-Rahe Stress Index[*]

Events	
Death of a spouse	100
Divorce	73
Marital separation	65
Jail term	63
Death of a close family member	63
Personal injury or illness	53
Marriage	50
Fired at work	47
Marital reconciliation	45
Retirement	45
Change in health of a family member	44
Pregnancy	40
Sexual difficulties	39
Gain of a new family member	39
Business readjustment	39
Change in financial state	38
Death of a close friend	37
Change to a different line of work	36
Change in number of arguments with spouse	35
Mortgage over $10,000	31

[*] Partial Listing

continues

Go ahead and measure your own stress score with the above events if they have occurred in the past year. If you score 150 or above, you have a 50 percent chance of illness or health change. If you score 300, you have a 90 percent chance of illness.

The point of this index is to make you aware of the stress level you may be under and yet may not realize. The above events occur in all of our lives, but interestingly not everyone becomes ill when they do occur. The researchers found that people who had the capability of "stress hardiness" had fewer illnesses connected to their stressful events.

How Can We Become Stress Hardy?

Dr. Suzanne Kobasa's research showed that stress hardiness can be cultivated by the three Cs: *challenges, control,* and *commitment.*[14]

Challenges

We know that stopping the challenges in our lives is impossible. The way to handle these events in our lives may be found in the words of Swami Satchitananda, "You can't stop the waves, but you can learn to surf."[15] Try to see problems as challenges, an opportunity to grow, rather than as a threat.

Control

Take control. Be proactive. The French word for coping comes from *coup,* a blow. It also means to strike back or to take control, so when we cope we are in control. Being proactive, rather than passive, and finding ways to take control helps us in coping with our stress. For my allergy and asthma patients, I recommend that in addition to monitoring their condition, they should do breathing exercises and yoga postures to help themselves regain some control.

Commitment

People who are committed to a group, whether it's their family, friends, or religious organizations, seem to have a greater capability to weather stressful events, disease, and even death. A classic study was done in 1979 by Lisa Berkman, an epidemiologist, and Leonard Syme, a professor at the University of California at Berkley. These researchers looked at the relationship between death rates and four types of social support: martial status, contact with extended family and friends, church membership, and other group affiliations. Their findings were quite amazing: people who were the least socially connected were twice as likely to die as those with the strongest social ties, even when health habits such as smoking, alcoholism, obesity, and exercise were taken into account.[16]

The type of questions you can ask yourself to see if you are isolated or more socially involved are:

> Do you live within twenty minutes of the same neighborhood where you were born and raised?
> Do you belong to a church or synagogue?
> Do you have family members within a short driving distance?
> If you were in an accident and hurt, do you have someone to go with you to the hospital?

Using the three Cs can prove invaluable in handling daily stress as well as long-term stresses, and you will find that as you become more "stress hardy," your allergies and asthma become steadily mitigated as well.

The best approach to becoming stress hardy is applying the three Cs with the mind-body techniques that are described in the next section.

Your Two-Step Daily Regimen for Relaxation and Stress Hardiness

Incorporating mind-body techniques into your daily life is as simple as breathing and remaining still for certain periods of time, and for this reason, anyone can achieve a healthy level of stress hardiness. The notion of some measure of time set aside every day strictly for relaxation is appealing to everyone—especially for those who will admit to stressful lifestyles—and with the promise of better health, there are no excuses to *not* treat yourself to a few moments of controlled R & R every day. What I prescribe is breath work, followed by yoga poses. In less than a half an hour a day, you can be well on your way to better health, lowered stress, and freedom from asthma.

Step 1: Breath Work

Many ancient cultures believed that the mind and the body are connected through the breath. While we all have to breathe to live, breath work, or conscious breathing, can be a bit more difficult than you might think. The mind is constantly inundated with thoughts, and this can distract you from relaxing. The way to quiet the mind is to focus on the breath.

Thich Nhat Hanh, a Buddhist monk and Nobel Peace Prize winner, has traveled the world and written many beautiful books teaching simple ways to conscious breathing and staying in the present moment—not worrying about the past or what will happen in the future.

One of my favorite exercises he teaches is:

> *Breathing in, I calm my body.*
> *Breathing out, I smile.*
> *Dwelling in the present moment,*
> *I know this is a wonderful moment!*[17]

The next set of breathing exercises and yoga I learned from Dr. Cristian Rachitan, who has traversed the globe studying these ancient techniques and teaching them to his patients. These exercises not only quiet the mind, but they also relax the spine and stretch the diaphragm muscle. The diaphragm is one of the largest muscles in the body, and it separates the body's upper organs (heart, lungs) from the lower organs (liver, spleen, intestines). It is the main muscle responsible for respiration. It is believed that stretching and activating this muscle sets a rhythm for internal organs to vibrate and work more effectively.

The breathing exercises should be done initially at least five days a week. And all it takes is fifteen minutes a day. This will get your mind and body into a rhythm, and you will see how the mind will struggle less with thoughts, and your expansion of your chest and belly will be greater. This will make it easier on your nose and chest breathing. Do these exercises in sequence for the best results.

To start your breathing exercises, it is important to find a quiet room in your home where you won't be disturbed. Early morning is a good time to do these exercises, as it gently gets the mind and body ready for the day's stressors. Phones and television should be turned off. You can play relaxing music preferably without words in the background. It's useful to have a small timer (such as a cooking timer) to regulate how much time you spend on a breathing exercise. These breathing exercises can be done while sitting in a chair with your back straight (not slouching) or on the floor in a cross-legged position, but your back should be supported by a wall. You should gently close your eyelids and let your eyes look upward at a 45 degree angle (this promotes a more relaxed rhythm of brain activity). Now you are ready for the first breath exercise.

Exercise 1: Lower Abdominal Breathing

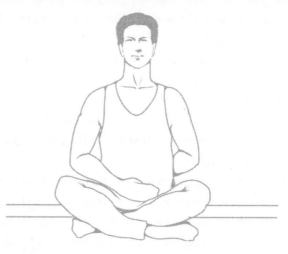

If you ever watch a baby breathe, you'll see her abdomen vibrating up and down. It's the natural way to use the abdominal muscles to help increase the lung capacity. As adults, we slowly lose this capacity, because our breathing becomes more constricted. This exercise will slowly help you regain your "belly breathing."

Deep breathing helps relax the lower spine. Sit comfortably in a straight-back chair or on the floor against a wall with your legs crossed. Place your left hand on your lower back and your right hand just below your navel. Begin by inhaling for four seconds with your abdomen protruding outward, and slowly allow the exhalation to flow through the nostrils for six seconds. Repeat this cycle again. Then, on every third breath, inhale for four seconds, hold the breath for six seconds, and then exhale for six seconds. Set a cooking timer for three minutes for this breathing exercise.

Exercise 2: Upper Chest Breathing

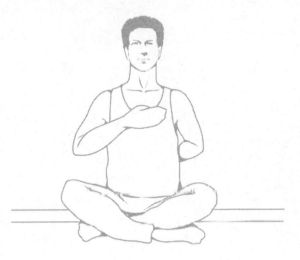

This exercise helps stretch the diaphragm. Start by placing your left hand high up behind your back, and your right hand in front of your chest over the *lower sternum* (where the ribs meet in front). Again, the cycle is to inhale for four seconds and exhale for six seconds, do it again, and then, on every third breath, inhale for four seconds, hold for six seconds, and then exhale slowly for six seconds. This exercise is also done for three minutes.

Exercise 3: Pumping Breathing

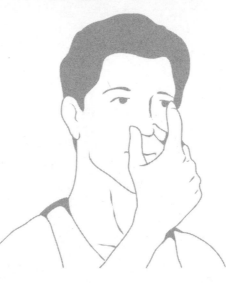

Seated in a chair or on the floor, place your right middle finger on your left nostril and your right thumb gently on your right nostril. Begin by forcefully exhaling through your nose, then breathe back in through one nostril and breathe back out through the opposite nostril. You can start with sets of ten, switching off between your left side and the right side. Don't go too fast, or you can get dizzy. This is one of the best exercises for loosening up the diaphragm. Caution: people with glaucoma (high eye pressure) and emphysema should avoid this exercise.

Exercise 4: Alternate Nostril Breathing

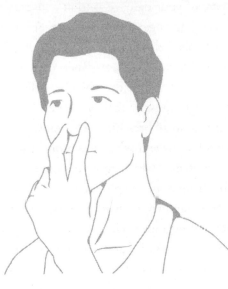

This last exercise is to be done very slowly. If done properly, it lets the air flow through the nostrils without any noise. You begin by placing your left index finger on your left nostril and inhaling through the right nostril for four seconds, then removing the left finger and allowing air to flow out the left nostril for six seconds. Then you inhale through the left nostril and exhale through the right nostril. You can start out doing this breathing exercise for three minutes and try to work up to six or eight minutes.

It's best to do the breathing exercises in the order in which they are presented. One of the things I've observed is that my patients who are professional singers (mainly opera) have tremendous ability to expand their chest and use their lung muscles when measuring their lung capacity. This is all from years of training—but you can learn it, too!

Step 2: Physical Exercises—Yoga Asanas

The second part of your daily relaxation consists of physical exercises that are based on yoga *asanas*, or poses. Some scientific reports have shown that yoga helps asthmatic patients.[18] It is also useful for pulmonary rehabilitation programs when used as physical therapy exercises to open and utilize the chest muscles. The diaphragm, which is the huge muscle that separates the chest from the abdomen, is critical in all breathing. This muscle easily tenses when a person is under stress and when the bronchioles get constricted. The breathing exercises, which relax and stretch only this muscle, make sense for this part of the program.

If you are not familiar with yoga exercises, I suggest you try taking a structured beginner's class at your local yoga studio, gym, or YMCA. Some community and spiritual centers also offer yoga, and it's helpful to have a bit of guidance before starting a new exercise program. You will also find it beneficial to visit your local library or bookstore and get an illustrated book on basic yoga poses to walk you through the following exercises. I found Esther Myers's book, *Yoga and You* very user-friendly.[19]

After your initial fifteen minutes of breathing exercises, you should spend at least fifteen minutes doing the following exercises to complete your daily relaxation routine. In the moments after you've completed your breathing exercises, your body is in a more relaxed state and is most receptive to the benefits of physical exercise or yoga asanas. You should be wearing loose-fitting clothing, as you don't want any restriction of movement, especially in the midsection from a belt. These exercises are intended to "lengthen" your body by stretching out your spine, hips, neck, abdomen—all the areas that are susceptible to the stress and tension of everyday life.

The physical exercises should be initially done at least five days a week to increase your body's flexibility. If you do them only infrequently and miss a few days in a row, your body tenses up again and you lose some of the prior gains of increased flexibility.

The first three groups of exercises that follow are a good way to begin your program to gently stretch and lengthen the body.

Phase 1: Standing Exercises
Mountain Pose

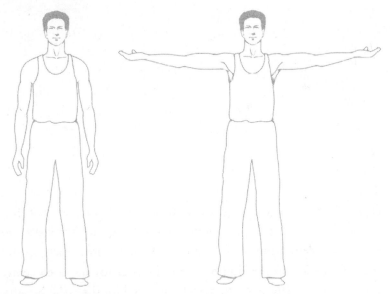

Begin this exercise by standing erect with your feet hip-width apart. Be aware of your weight being transmitted down your legs to your feet. Feel the contact of your heels with the floor. Focus on your breath and feel your belly moving back and forth. Slowly raise your arms until they are extended out 90 degrees on both sides. Hold your arms like this for three breaths. Next, begin to raise your arms so they are 180 degrees above your sides. Now, interlace your index fingers pointing upward. Hold this position for three full breaths. Slowly lower your arms down to your sides.

Half Moon

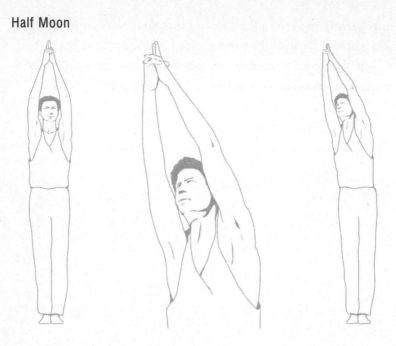

Begin this exercise by raising your arms overhead. Interlace your fingers with your index fingers pointed upward. Keeping the waist and lower body firm, bend to the right. At the same time reach up and outward. Hold this position for three full breaths, and then center yourself again. Now, bend to the left and hold for three full breaths. Come back to the center position and slowly release your arms to your sides.

Spinal Breath

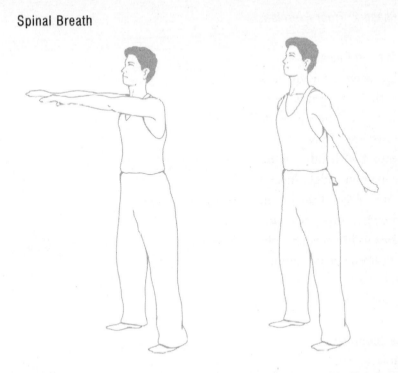

Standing up straight with your arms at your sides, take three full breaths. Raise your arms in front of you and exhale forcefully. On the *in-breath,* bring your arms all the way behind your body. Hold that position for three breaths, and then bring your arms in front again. Repeat this exercise two more times.

Phase 2: Floor Exercises

Knee to Chest

Lie down on your back with your knees bent and feet firmly pressing into the floor. Clasp your two hands behind your right thigh. Take a nice deep breath in. Slowly, on the *out-breath,* bring your right leg up by gently pulling the back of your thigh. Go as far as is comfortable to you. Holding this position for ten seconds.

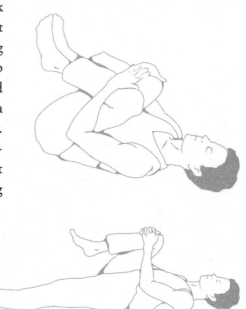

(Don't forget to continue your breathing.) Now, slowly inhale as you release your leg back to the floor. Next, repeat this exercise with your left leg. After you have done both legs individually, bring both legs up to the chest and hold this position for ten seconds (of course, don't forget the breathing). *The benefit of this exercise is that it releases the lower back and lengthens the spine; this is very safe and helps people with lower back problems.*

Trunk Twist

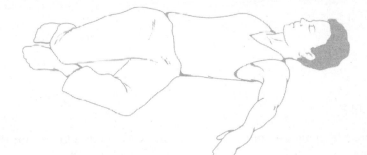

Lie on your back with your knees bent and feet firmly pressing into the floor. Keep your arms extended out at your sides. Take a deep breath in, and on the *out-breath*, allow your knees to fall slowly to your right side, as far as your hips will allow you to twist. Hold this position for ten seconds, and continue to breathe in and out. Then bring yourself back to your original position. Now, allow your legs to fall to your left side and hold this position. Return your knees to the middle and take three full breaths.

Bridge Pose

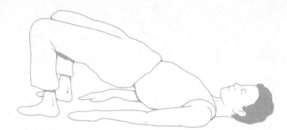

Start by lying on your back with your knees bent and feet on the floor, hip-width apart. Your lower back should be flat against the floor. Focus on your abdominal breathing for a few seconds. On the *in-breath*, slowly and gently elevate your buttocks a few inches off the floor, and then slowly let them touch the floor on the *out-breath*. On the next inhalation, raise your buttocks up as high as is comfortable. Try to hold this position for three full breaths, and then exhale slowly on the way down.

Pelvic Tilt

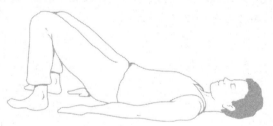

Lie on the floor with your knees bent and feet hip-width apart. Take your hand and feel for the space between the arch of your lower back against the floor. On the *in-breath*, feel your belly rise, and on the *out-breath*, as your belly collapses, press your lower back into the floor so that it lies flush against the floor. Hold this position for three relaxation breaths and then release.

Phase 3: Kneeling Exercises

Cat Position

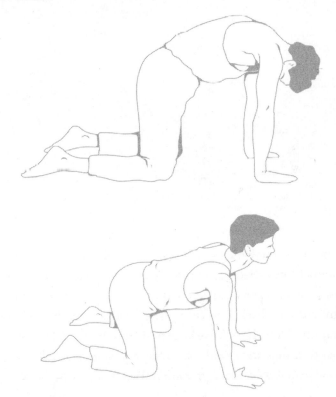

Start on your hands and knees, with your hands underneath your shoulders and your knees underneath your hips. Exhaling, curl your pelvis under and press down with the heels of your hand to round your back. Let your head drop. As you inhale, relax your spine and allow your belly to gently hang. Hold this position for three breaths, and then repeat the exhalation motion slowly. Alternate these movements for a dynamic and relaxing release of the spine.

Prayer Pose

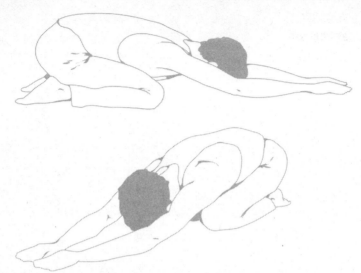

Begin again on your hands and knees, and slowly sit back. If possible, your buttocks are pressing against the heels of your feet. Bend forward and rest your arms and head on the floor. As you exhale, let your hips drop toward your heels, and continue your relaxation breathing for three breaths. Note: if you have knee problems, place a folded blanket between your hips and your heels. *This position is an excellent way to stretch out the lower back and get into a relaxed mental state.*

By making time for breathing exercises and yoga every day, you are taking a critical step toward better stress and asthma management. You will likely notice that even before you notice how much healthier and revitalized your body feels, these quiet moments offer you a welcomed escape from the travails of daily life. This two-step program will prove to be an escape that you never knew you needed. But as doing these exercises in times of stress becomes second nature to you, you will wonder how you ever did without them.

CHAPTER

12

Five Steps to Becoming Allergy Free

I was taught from grade school through medical school that achieving anything worthwhile takes a lot of hard work. The good news is that, in many cases, hard work pays off. The first four steps of this program are in your hands and its success depends on your diligence. The final step involves a cooperative effort with your physician to achieve a life where allergies no longer interfere with life.

Step 1: Become an Educated Patient

Medicine has changed. Pharmaceutical companies can market drugs directly to the public through the media, using television, radio, and magazines. They do it very effectively. The public does become more aware of the new products that are available. However, knowing specific facts without having the proper bank of knowledge to ground them can sometimes be a dangerous thing. I strongly urge you to not take the pharmaceutical companies' advertising claims at face value.

The Internet offers many opportunities for patients to find out all about the different treatment modalities that are available. You can learn more about conventional and holistic treatments, as well as complementary treatments (the combination of both). Three Internet sites that provide reliable information about treatment are the American College of Allergy, Asthma, and Immunology site (www.ACAI.org.), the American Academy of Allergy, Asthma, and Immunology site (www.AAAAI.org), and the American Academy of Otolaryngology Allergy site (www.AAOA.org). I also highly recommend the Allergy Choices Web site (www.Allergychoices.com), where you can learn more about the sublingual allergy method of treatment.

My own Web site, www.AllergyDrops.net, shows patients what it is like to visit my office and provides information on the latest developments in the field of allergy. The value of being an educated medical consumer is huge. It puts you in the driver's seat. You now have the ability to get information and make choices based on available options.

Step 2: Eliminate or Avoid Your Allergens

If your fiancé brings you a guinea pig as a present and two weeks later you notice you are always short of breath and itch a lot, ask him to find the guinea pig a new home right away. If you are in a long-term relationship with your cat or dog when you first become allergic to it and can't bring yourself to send your pet away, even though you understand the cause of your problem, please follow these rules:

1. Keep pets out of your bedroom and off your bed. If they sleep in your room, you will be inhaling their dander all

night long. When you are sleeping, your body doesn't clear your secretions as well, so putting yourself in this response-provoking situation can lead to severe respiratory symptoms.

2. Buy a reliable air-filtration device. It will remove some of the dander particles in the air.

3. Wash your pet at least once a week, or if this is too impractical, wipe your pet down with a damp washcloth to keep the dander from fluffing up and getting into the air.

If you suffer from dust allergies, you should encase your mattress and pillowcases in protective covers that trap the dust mites and kill them and wash your sheets in hot water every week to remove the mites. You should also monitor the humidity in your home with a hygrometer purchased at a hardware store. If the humidity in the room is over 50 percent, you should purchase a dehumidifier that can lower it to below 30 percent. Since dust mites don't thrive in low-humidity environments, they won't be provoking your allergies and asthma as much, and your condition will improve. If your home is moldy and damp, you should also consider getting dehumidifiers so that the mold can't thrive.

And finally, eliminate any cockroaches. If, heaven forbid, your home is infested with them, check the Yellow Pages for a good exterminator and rid yourself of this potent allergen. Allergy Control Products, Inc. (www.AllergyControl.com) and National Allergy Supply, Inc. (www.NationalAllergySupply.com) are two fine and reputable companies that offer quality products for environmental control. They also have very qualified representatives available by telephone to suggest what products might be best for you and your home.

Step 3: Be Proactive in Your Health
You can do this in two ways. First, record in your journal, daily

calendar, or blackberry how you are feeling. It's simple: on a scale of one to ten (ten meaning your feel great and are without symptoms) put down in your log at the end of each day how you feel symptomwise for a month, or during a period when you know you have difficulty. This helps you and your doctor see if there is a pattern to your symptoms and let's you become aware if your are improving. Second, don't just sit there, do something! In reading this book, I'm sure you can tell that I'm a strong advocate of taking personal control of your health. A doctor can recommend all the textbook steps, but if a patient doesn't follow them, what good are they? But even more important, there is a wealth of information about how stress plays a huge role in all illnesses, and it seems this is something that can't be cured with a pill. That's why I advocate using the Better Breathing Program described in chapter 11 that involves breathing techniques, yoga, and group support. You might have to be a little creative to put together a program, but here are some suggestions:

1. Join a local YMCA. Many now offer yoga classes, and most yoga classes offer some type of breathing exercises.
2. Check with your local hospital. Many of them now offer alternative medicine programs with meditation, yoga, and helpful nutritional advice.
3. Join a support group for people with allergies and asthma. As I mentioned, the Food Allergy Network has meetings and frequent online advice. Mothers for Asthmatics is another excellent source of information, and usually your local hospital has programs. I can't emphasize enough how important group support is. I'll repeat a favorite line from Dr. Bernie Siegel: "The doctor is the tourist, the patient is the native," which means

patients know things a doctor may never feel—and only another patient can give you the support that can heal you.

Step 4: Be Careful about What You Eat

We have discussed the ways that food can affect your allergies. Know which foods can trigger yours, and become a good label reader! When you eat out at restaurants, warn your waiter that certain foods give you allergic reactions and list them for him. Make sure that he tells the chef so that in the kitchen they'll take care to avoid bringing your food into contact with someone else's dish (which may contain something you are allergic to.) If you have food allergies, remember that raw foods provoke more allergic responses than cooked foods, and watch out for the foods that cross-react with your pollen allergies (as discussed in chapter 10.) Become an educated consumer and join the Food Allergy Network. Keep a food diary. My wife, Dr. Ricki Mitchell, is a medical nutritionist. She always urges her patients to keep a food diary, and she is right! A food diary makes you proactive in assessing your help. Ricki and I ask our patients to record what they eat for a week on a grid sheet that separates breakfast, lunch, and dinner and has spaces for snacks. There is also a section for symptoms. This achieves two things: (1) it allows the patient to be more cognizant of what they are actually eating—for example, "Oh, my, I've been eating cheese everyday," and (2) it allows the doctor to see if there are certain foods that may be aggravating a patient's symptoms (remember the All-American Sandwich Story). When patients are vested in their treatment plans, they will work harder and most likely will get better results.

Weekly Food Diary

		Day #1	Day #2	Day #3	Day #4	Day #5	Day #6	Day #7
Time 8 AM – 11 AM	**BREAKFAST** FOODS Specific: Cereals Brands BEVERAGES Specific: Milk Coffee Tea							
Time	Symptoms							
	Medication							
1 PM – 3 PM	**LUNCHEON** FOODS Specific: Candy BEVERAGES Specific: Soda							
Time	Symptoms							
	Medication							
6 PM – 8 PM	**DINNER** FOODS Specific: BEVERAGES Specific: Snacks							
Time	Symptoms							
	Medication							

Step 5: See Your Doctor . . . Don't Be Your Own Doctor

If trying all the above steps has not brought you the relief you are seeking, then it's important to take the final and possibly most important step: selecting a doctor who can help you diagnose and treat your allergies. If you diagnose yourself and your conclusions are incorrect (which is certainly a possibility), anything you do after that only delays your getting proper treatment. During your first visit to the doctor, a proper medical history will be taken and you'll have a physical exam. This can give your doctor some clues whether you have underlying allergies. But the only way to know for sure is to get tested! The ImmunoCap allergy blood test will tell you and your doctor specific allergies. Then treatment can be targeted to your problem.

If your general doctor or pediatrician has not been able to help you as much as you need, you should ask to see an allergist, who is specially trained to recognize and treat allergic conditions. Almost all insurance companies cover visits to allergists as well as the testing they do to establish the facts about your condition. My main advice about seeing an allergist is that you should also become an active participant in your care. When the doctor tells you exactly what you are allergic to, *write it all down!* If you need allergy immunotherapy, *find out exactly what your vaccine is made of.* Ask questions! If you live in New York City, you shouldn't need horsehair in your vaccine (unless you operate a horse-drawn carriage in Central Park).

If you have asthma, ask your doctor to write an Asthma Action Plan for you. As you have seen in the example in our book, you need to be a partner in this enterprise, and record your peak flow readings every day. After you have done this for two to four weeks, show your records to your doctor. They will indicate whether you are improving and help the doctor decide if your medication should be adjusted. Remember, the first key step is to control your asthma, then hopefully you can move on to the reversal phase!

Finally, if you have tried prescription and nonprescription medicines without getting any relief, if you have implemented the necessary environmental controls but are still suffering, if you can't avoid your close friend's cat or dog though this provokes your allergies, or if you can't play golf in the spring because of your reactions to the season, you are a good candidate for sublingual allergy immunotherapy, the "allergy drops." The goal of this therapy is the reversal of your allergies, which should bring you to a better quality of life. It is should also decrease or eliminate your need for medication. It is not a therapy that must be prolonged for a lifetime. After a few years you should be better and no longer need treatment.

I'm sure that *Dr. Dean Mitchell's Allergy and Asthma Solution* will not be the last word in this exciting field, but I hope you will find it useful in your journey toward relief from your allergies and asthma. As the driving partner in your own health care, you are taking the steps necessary to ensure better health and well-being— for yourself and for your loved ones.

Acknowledgments

This book has been a labor of love in many ways. It has given me the chance to share the exciting new breakthrough treatment of sublingual allergy immunotherapy and at the same time to reflect on the many success stories of my own patients.

But first I have to thank my agent, Carol Mann, for taking a chance on an unknown doctor who "cold-called" her, and FOR believing in this new treatment. I would also like to thank Matthew Lore and Avalon Publishing for making this book a reality. It is with great appreciation that I would like to thank Renée Sedliar, my editor at Marlowe & Company, for her insightful comments and support. In addition, Mari Florence and Laurie Bernstein helped guide me in editing early versions of the book. I also appreciate the early support and encouragement from Caroline Gregorio and Stacey Sharaby.

You can become an experienced physician only if you see many cases. I want to express my appreciation to colleagues of mine who supported my choice to follow a new path. Dr. Michael Gnatt, a superb physician who combines alternative medicine with modern technology, has been a true friend and was an early supporter of my work. For their friendship and support I also thank Dr. Maria Musso and Dr. Joseph Tarrantino, as well as the following colleagues: David Pearl, Carol Larson, Richard Amiraian, Kelly Cassano, Linda Attoe, Tony Flanders, Betty Parisis, Neil Soskel, Ron Falcon, Mary Jenkins, Sue Nadeson, John Wang, John Olichney, Gae Rodke, and Lawrence and Albert Attia. A special thanks goes to Dr. James Dillard for his advice on how to become a physician-author. I would also like to thank Paul Barth at the Roosevelt Hospital Medical Library for his help in obtaining many articles I used to learn about sublingual immunotherapy.

A physician in today's world can only survive with the help of a great staff. I would like to thank Maria Centurion for her adroitness in handling our busy New York City practice and for her exceptional skill in helping me make correction after correction so that each draft came out just right. I want to thank my longtime nurse, Mildred Weaver, for her faith that this project would come to fruition and for helping me care for and train countless patients in the proper use of the allergy drops. My other staff members, Pat Nicosia, Gladys Castano, and Lynne Scheinin, made practicing fun again by running such an efficient practice on Long Island.

Every doctor has role models he or she looks up to, who inspire him or her to be the best they can be. Dr. David Morris and his partners, Mary Morris, George Kroker, and Vijay Sabnis, were all so helpful, and great teachers, when I first began to introduce sublingual allergy immunotherapy into my practice.

In my own backyard, New York, there are a number of doctors who I believe fit the "gold standard," because they represent everything that you want in a doctor; they are smart, kind, caring, and open to new developments. Dr. Nicholas Macris has for forty years trained allergists at Lenox Hill and Cornell's Allergy Fellowship.

He is unparalleled in his skill and knowledge and is one of the true allergist-immunologists to ever practice. Dr. Vincent Beltrani, one of only a few dual board-certified allergist-dermatologists, was an exceptional teacher when I rotated through Columbia's dermatology clinic, and his pearls of wisdom and effervescent personality have inspired me to be a better doctor. I also want to thank Marty Mongione, who provided sound advice on the Asthma Action Plan and helped initiate me into the world of computer technology. Also, for their excellent work in supplying the drawings for the book: Justin Marler for the medical drawings and Kajiah Jacobs for the yoga and breathing drawings.

And finally, inspiration may come from within, but it sure helps to have a lot of support at home. My parents, Mitch and Gloria Mitchell, have always been there for me through life's up and downs, and have instilled in me the belief that dreams can come true. My wife, Ricki, has been my staunchest advocate. It's nice to have a wife who's as smart as a doctor can get, and with whom you can discuss anything from an allergy case to our children's homework in the same sentence, without missing a beat. And to my two precious boys, Zach and Stone—thanks for letting your dad finish his "homework" for the past four years.

Notes

Chapter 1: What Are Allergies?

1. L. M. Fromer, "Clinical Rationale for Obtaining a Precise Diagnosis." *The Journal of Family Practice,* supplement April 2004, S4–S14.

2. K. Ishizaka, and T. Ishizaka, "Identification of Gamma-E Antibodies as a Carrier of Reagenic Activity," *Journal of Immunology* 99 (1967): 1187–98.

3. F. D. Martinez, et al., "Asthma and Wheezing in the First Six Years of Life," *New England Journal of Medicine* 332 (1995): 133–8.

4. A. Simpson, L. Soderstrom, S. Ahlstedt, "IgE Antibody Quantification and the Probability of Wheeze in Preschool Children." *J Allergy Clin Immunol,* 116, no. 4 (October 2005): 744–9.

5. G. J. Gleich, "Mechanisms of Eosinophil-Associated Inflammation," *Journal of Allergy and Clinical Immunology* 105 (2000): 651–3.

6. Ibid.

7. W. W. Busse, and R. F. Lemanske, "Advances in Immunology: Asthma," *New England Journal of Medicine* 344 (2001): 350–62.

Chapter 2: Why Are Allergies So Prevalent Today?

1. S. J. Arbes, P. J. Gergen, L. Elliot, D. C. Zeldin, "Prevalences of Positive Skin Test Responses to 10 Common Allergens in the U.S. Population: Results from the Third National Health and Nutrition Examination Survey." *J Allergy Clin Immunol*, 116, no. 2 (August 2005): 377–83.

2. T. A. Platts-Mills and J. A. Woodfolk, "Rise in Asthma Cases," *Science* 278 (1997): 1001.

3. P. R. Epstein, "Climate Changes Change and Human Health," *New England Journal of Medicine* 353 (2005).

4. R. W. Weber, "Mother Nature Strikes Back: Global Warming, Homeostasis, and Implications for Allergy," *Annals of Allergy, Asthma, and Immunology* 88 (2002): 251–2.

5. J. A. Bernstein, et al., "Health Effects of Air Pollution," *Journal of Allergy and Clinical Immunology* 114 (2004): 1116–23.

6. Ibid.

7. P. H. Ryan, et al., "Is It Traffic Type, Volume or Distance? Wheezing in Infants Living Near Truck and Bus Traffic." *J Allergy Clin Immunol* 116 (2005): 279–84.

8. T. A. Platts-Mills, et al., "Indoor Allergens and Asthma: Report of the Third International Workshop," *Journal of Allergy and Clinical Immunology* 100 (1997): S2–24.

9. L. R. Skadhauge, K. Christensen, K. O. Kyvik, and T. Sigsgaard, "Genetic and Environmental Influence on Asthma: A Population-Based Study of 11,688 Danish Twin Pairs," *European Respiratory Journal* 13 (1999): 8–14.

10. International Study of Asthma and Allergies in Childhood (ISAAC) Steering Committee, "Worldwide Variation in Prevalence of Symptoms of Asthma, Allergic Rhinoconjunctivitis, and Atopic Eczema: ISAAC," *Lancet* 351 (1998): 1225–32.

11. J. Mattes, et al., "The Use of Antibiotics in the First Year of Life and

Development of Asthma: Which Comes First?" *Clinical and Experimental Allergy* 29 (1999): 729–32.

12. S. T. Weiss, "Eat Dirt—The Hygiene Hypothesis and Allergic Disease." *N Engl J Med* 347, no. 2 (2002): 930–1.

13. T. M. Ball, et al., "Siblings, Day-Care Attendance, and the Risk of Asthma and Wheezing during Childhood," *New England Journal of Medicine* 343 (2000): 538–43.

14. S. O. Shaheen, et al., "Measles and Atopy in Guinea-Bissau," *Lancet* 347 (1996): 1792–6.

15. D. P. Strachan, "Hay Fever, Hygiene, and Household Size," *British Medical Journal* 299 (1989): 1259–60.

16. C. Braun-Fahrlander, J. Riedler, U. Herz, "Environmental Exposure to Endotoxin and its relation to asthma in school-age children." *N Engl J Med* 347, no. 12 (2002): 869–79.

Chapter 3: The Allergic Evaluation: It Doesn't Have to Hurt!

1. R. G. Hamilton, and N. F. Adkinson, Jr., "In vitro Assays for the Diagnosis of IgE-Mediated Disorders," *Journal of Allergy and Clinical Immunology* 114 (2004): 213–25.

2. R. G. Roberts, "Seeking IgE—Know the Allergen, Improve the Care," *Patient Care* 38 (2004): 28–33.

3. G. Shepherd, M. Betancourt, "What's in the Air?" *Pocket Books* (2002): 100–3.

4. H. A. Sampson, "Can We Diagnose Atopy with a Laboratory Test?" *Annals of Allergy, Asthma, and Immunology* 93 (2004): 307–08.

5. A. Fiocchi, R. Besana, A. Ryden, et al., "Differential Diagnosis of IgE-Mediated Allergy in Young Children with Wheezing or Eczema Symptoms Using a Single Blood Test," *Annals of Allergy, Asthma, and Immunology* 93 (2004): 328–32.

Chapter 4: What Are the Standard Treatments for Allergies and Asthma?

1. W. D. Finkle, J. L. Adams, S. Greenland, and K. L. Melmon, "Increased Risk of Serious Injury Following an Initial Prescription for Diphenhydramine," *Annals of Allergy, Asthma, and Immunology* 89 (2002): 244–50.

2. J. C. Verster, and E. R. Volkerts, "Antihistamines and Driving Ability: Evidence from On-the-Road Driving Studies During Normal Traffic," *Annals of Allergy, Asthma, and Immunology* 92 (2004): 294–303.

3. B. Q. Lanier, J. Corren, W. Lumry, et al., "Omalizumab Is Effective in the Long-term Control of Severe Allergic Asthma," *Annals of Allergy, Asthma, and Immunology* 91 (2003): 154–9.

4. M. Cabana, et al., "Parental Management of Asthma Triggers within a Child's Environment," *Journal of Allergy and Clinical Immunology* 114 (2004): 352–7.

5. L. G. Arlian, J. S. Neal, and D. L. Vyszenski-Moher, "Reducing Relative Humidity to Control the House Dust Mite Dermatophagoides farinae," *Journal of Allergy and Clinical Immunology* 104 (1999): 852–6.

6. P. Cabrera, G. Julia-Serda, F. Rodriguez de Castro, et al., "Reduction of House Dust Mite Allergens after Dehumidifier Use," *Journal of Allergy and Clinical Immunology* 95 (1995): 635–6.

7. *Consumer Reports* "Ionizing Air Cleaners," May 2005, cosumerreports.org.

8. C. M. Luczynski, Y. Li, M. D. Chapman, and T. A. Platts-Mills, "Airborne Concentration and Particle Size Distribution of Allergen Derived from Domestic Cats (Felis domesticus). Measurements Using Cascade Impactor, Liquid Impinger and a Two-site Monoclonal Antibody Assay for Fel d 1," *American Review of Respiratory Disease* 141 (1990): 361–7.

9. J. W. Vaughan, J. A. Woodfolk, and T. A. Platts-Mills, "Assessment of Vacuum Cleaners and Vacuum Cleaner Bags Recommended for

Allergic Subjects," *Journal of Allergy and Clinical Immunology* 104 (1999): 1079–83.

10. D. L. Rosenstreich, P. Eggleston, M. Kattan, et al., "The Role of Cockroach Allergen in Causing Morbidity Among Inner-city Children with Asthma," *New England Journal of Medicine* 336 (1997): 1356–63.

11. W. J. Morgan, E. F. Crain, and R. S. Gruchalla, et al., "Results of a Home-based Environmental Intervention Among Urban Children with Asthma," *New England Journal of Medicine* 351 (2004): 1068–80.

Chapter 5: The Concept of Allergy Immunotherapy

1. S. R. Durham, et al., "Immunological Changes Associated with Allergen Immunotherapy," *Journal of Allergy and Clinical Immunology* 102 (1998): 157–64.

2. F. E. Simons, *Ancestors of Allergy* (New York: Global Medical Communications, 1994).

3. R. F. Lockey, S. G. Burkantz, and J. Bosquetsa, *Allergens and Allergy Immunotherapy*, p. 23, 3rd ed. (Marcæl Dekker: 2004).

4. Samuel Hahnemann, *Organon of Medicine*, 6th ed. (1842).

5. D. L. Morris, "Intradermal Testing and Sublingual Desensitization for Nickel," *Cutis* 61 (1998): 129–32.

Chapter 6: No More Shots! Sublingual Allergy Immunotherapy

1. R. F. Lockey, L. M. Benedict, et al., "Fatalities from Immunotherapy and Skin Testing," *Journal of Allergy and Clinical Immunology* 79 (1987): 660.

2. J. F. Schamberg, "Desensitization of Persons against Poison Ivy," *Journal of the American Medical Association* 73 (1919): 1213.

3. R. Clavel, J. Bousquet, and C. Andre, "Clinical Efficacy of Sublingual-Swallow Immunotherapy: A Double-Blind, Placebo-Controlled Trial of Standardized Five-Grass-Pollen Extract in Rhinitis," *Allergy* 53 (1998): 493–98.

4. C. Andre, C. Vatrinet, S. Galvain, et al., "Safety of Sublingual-Swallow Immunotherapy in Children and Adults," *International Archives of Allergy and Applied Immunology* 121 (2000): 229–34.

5. E. J. Van Wilsen, "Dendritic Cells of the Oral Mucosa and the Induction of Oral Tolerance: A Local Affair," *Immunology* 83 (1994): 128–32.

6. J. Bousquet, R. Lockey, and H. Malling, "WHO Position Paper: Allergy Immunotherapy: Therapeutic Vaccines for Allergic Disease," *Allergy* 53, Supplement (1998): S54.

7. C. Andre, C. Vatrinet, S. Galvain, et al., "Safety of Sublingual-Swallow Immunotherapy in Children and Adults," *International Archives of Allergy and Applied Immunology* 121 (2000): 229–34.

8. V. Feliziani, G. Lattuada, S. Parmiani, et al., "Safety and Efficacy of Sublingual Rush Immunotherapy with Grass Allergen Extracts: A Double-Blind Study," *Allergologia et Immunopathologia* (Madrid) 23 (1995): 224–30.

9. T. Bowen et al., "Canadian Trial of Sublingual Swallow Immunotherapy for Ragweed Rhinoconjunctivitis." *Annals of Allergy, Asthma & Immunology* 93 (November 2004): 425–30.

10. Margona M, Spadolini I, Massolo A, et al., "Randomized Controlled Open Study of Sublingual Immunotherapy (SLIT) for Respiratory Allergy in Real Life: Clinical Efficacy and More." *Allergy* 59 (2004): 1205-10.

11. G. W. Canonica, and G. Passalacqua, "Noninjection Routes of Immunotherapy," *Journal of Allergy and Clinical Immunology* 111 (2003): 437–48.

12. C. Lombardi, F. Gani, M. Landi, et al., "Quantitative Assessment of the Adherence to Sublingual Immunotherapy," *Journal of Allergy and Clinical Immunology* 113 (2004): 1219–20.

13. T. Lower, J. Henry, et al., "Compliance with Allergen Immunotherapy," *Annals of Allergy, Asthma, and Immunology* 70 (1993): 480–82.

14. D. Tinkelman, et al., "Compliance with an Allergen Immunotherapy Regime," *Annals of Allergy, Asthma, and Immunology* 74 (1995): 241–6.

15. B. Rhodes, "Patient Dropouts before Completion of Optimal Dose, Multiple-Allergen Immunotherapy," *Annals of Allergy, Asthma, and Immunology* 82 (1999): 281–6.

16. J. R. Cohn, and A. Pizzi, "Determinants of Patient Compliance with Allergen Immunotherapy," *Journal of Allergy and Clinical Immunology* 91 (1993): 734–7.

17. S. R. Durham, S. M. Walker, et al., "Long-term Clinical Efficacy of Grass-Pollen Immunotherapy," *New England Journal of Medicine* 341 (1999): 468–75.

Chapter 7: The Asthma Action Plan

1. W. W. Busse, and R. F. Lemanske, "Advances in Immunology: Asthma," *New England Journal of Medicine* 344 (2001): 350–62.

2. M. Schatz, C. Sorkness, James Li, et al., "Asthma Control Test: Reliability, Validity, and Responsiveness in Patients Not Previously Followed by Asthma Specialists." *J Allergy Clin Immunol*, 117, no. 3, (2006): 549–51.

3. National Heart, Lung and Blood Institute. NAEEP Expert Panel Report, Guidelines for the Diagnosis and Management of Asthma—Update on Selected Topics 2002. Bethesda, MD.

4. Timothy H. Self, Kimberlee E. Kilgore, Victor Shelton, "Pitfalls in Prescibing: MDI's—Spacers and Dry Powder Inhalers: What Patients Are Likely to Do Wrong." *Consultant* (May 2003): 702–5.

5. Fernando D. Martinez. "Safety of Long-acting Beta-Agonists—An Urgent Need to Clear the Air." *N Engl J Med* 353: 2637–9.

6. V. D. Rienzo, F. Marcucci, et al, "Long-lasting Effect of Sublingual Immunotherapy in Children with Asthma Due to House Mite: A 10 Year Prospective Study." *Clin Exp Allergy* 23 (2003): 206–10.

7. Jeffrey Kluger, "Asthma Alarm: Millions of Kids Would Breathe Easier If Their Parents Paid Closer Attention," *Time* 164 (December 20, 2004): 162.

8. F. D. Martinez, et al., "Asthma and Wheezing in the First Six Years of Life," *New England Journal of Medicine* 332 (1995): 133–8.

9. R. Sporik, et al., "Mite, Cat, and Cockroach Exposure, Allergen Sensitization, and Asthma in Children: A Case-control Study of Three Schools," *Thorax* 54 (1999): 675–80.

10. D. L. Rosenstreich, et al., "The Role of Cockroach Allergy and Exposure to Cockroach Allergen in Causing Morbidity Among Inner-city Children with Asthma," *New England Journal of Medicine* 336 (1997): 1356–63.

11. M. T. O'Hallaren, J. W. Yunginger, K. P. Offord, et al., "Exposure to an Aeroallergen as a Possible Precipitating Factor in Respiratory Arrest in Young Patients with Asthma." *N Engl J Med* 234 (1991): 359–63.

12. Theresa W. Guilbert, Wayne J. Morgan, Robert S. Zeiger, et al., "Atopic Characteristics of Children with Recurrent Wheezing at High Risk for the Development of Childhood Asthma," *Journal of Allergy and Clinical Immunology* 114., no 6 (2004): 1282–7.

13. A. Simpson, L. Soderstrom, S. Ahlstedt, "IgE Antibody Quantification and the Probability of Wheeze in Preschool Children." *J Allergy Clin Immunol*, 116, no. 4 (October 2005): 744–9.

14. Elio Novembre, Elena galli, Fabio Landi, et al., "Co-seasonal Sublingual ImmunoTherapy Reduces the Development of Asthma in Children with Allergic Rhinoconjunctivitis," *J Allergy Clin Immunol*, (October 2004): 851–7.

Chapter 8: Diseases That Masquerade as Allergies or Asthma . . . but Aren't

1. K. G. Lim, and T. I. Morgenthaler, "Pulmonary Function Tests, Part 1: Applying the Basics," *Journal of Respiratory Diseases* 26 (2005): 26–39.

2. A. Abidov, A. Rozanski, R. Hachamovitch, et al., "Prognostic Significance of Dyspnea in Patients Referred for Cardiac Stress Testing," *New England Journal of Medicine* 353 (2005): 1889–98.

3. Peter McNally, *GI/Liver Secrets*, 2nd ed. (Philadelphia: Hanley and Belfus, 2001).

4. R. C. Balkisson, "Difficult to Manage Asthma: Is it Vocal Cord Dysfunction?" *Clinical Courier*, 23, no. 32 (August 2005):. 5–6.

5. E. Eden, D. Mitchell, et al., Atopy, "Asthma and Emphysema in Patients with Severe Alpha-1-Antitrypsin Deficiency," *American Journal of Respiratory and Critical Care Medicine* 156 (1997): 68–74.

6. John A. Elliot, *Case Presentations in Respiratory Medicine* (London: Butterworths, 1999).

7. Laura Inselman, *Pediatric Pulmonary Pearls* (Philadelphia: Hanley and Belfus, 2001).

8. Bruce Jafek and Bruce Murrow, *ENT Secrets*, 2nd ed. (Philadelphia: Hanley and Belfus, 2001).

Chapter 9: Chronic Sinus Disease and the New Research

1. M. A. Kaliner, et al., "Sinusitis: Bench to Bedside. Current Findings, Future Directions," *Journal of Allergy and Clinical Immunology* 99 (1997): S829–48.

2. L. Borish, "Chronic Hyperplastic Eosinophilic Sinusitis," Lecture Series, Medical College of Georgia, 2001.

3. J. U. Ponikau, et al., "The Diagnosis and Incidence of Allergic Fungal Sinusitis," *Mayo Clinic Proceedings* 74 (1999): 877–84.

4. I. Emmanuel and S. Shah, "Chronic rhinosinustis: Allergy and Sinus Computed Tomography Relationship." *Otolaryngol Head Neck Surg*, 123, no. 6 (December 2000): 687–91 December 2000.

5. J. H. Krouse, "Computed Tomography Stage, Allergy Testing, and Quality of Life in Patients with Sinusitis." *Otolaryngol Head Neck Surg* 123 (2000): 389-92.

6. Jane E. Brody, "When Trouble Hits Those Holes in Your Head." *NY Times,* Tuesday March 15, 2005.
7. D. D. Stevenson, et al., "Aspirin Desensitization Treatment of Aspirin-sensitive Patients with Rhinosinusitis-Asthma: Long-term Outcomes," *Journal of Allergy and Clinical Immunology* 98 (1996): 751–8.
8. Dr. Andrew Weil's Self-Healing, "Seven Strategies for Sinus Relief." November 2005, pg.1

Chapter 10: Food Allergies
1. "Research Update: Advances in the Past Year." *Food Allergy News* 14, no. 3 (February–March 2005): 1–5.
2. S. A. Bock, H. A. Sampson, F. M. Atkins, et al., "Double-Blind, Placebo-Controlled Food Challenge (DBPCFC) as an Office Procedure: A Manual," *Journal of Allergy and Clinical Immunology* 82 (1988): 986–7.
3. H. A. Sampson, "Fatal Food-Induced Anaphylaxis," *Allergy* 53 (1998): 125–30.
4. M. M. Rawas-Qalaji, F. E. Simons, and K. J. Simons, "Sublingual Epinephrine Tablets Versus Intramuscular Injection of Epinephrine: Dose Equivalence for Potential Treatment of Anaphylaxis," *Journal of Allergy and Clinical Immunology* 117, no. 2, (2006): 398–403.
5. D. Y. Leung, H. A. Sampson, J. W. Yunginger, et al., "Effect of Anti-IgE Therapy in Patients with Peanut Allergy," *New England Journal of Medicine* 348 (2003): 986–93.
6. K. D. Srivastava, J. D. Kattan, Z. M. Zou, et al., "The Chinese Herbal Medicine Formula FAHF-2 Completely Blocks Anaphylactic Reactions in a Murine Model of Peanut Allergy," *Journal of Allergy and Clinical Immunology* 115 (2005): 171–8.
7. E. Enrique, F. Pineda, et al., "Sublingual Immunotherapy for Hazelnut Food Allergy: A Randomized, Double-Blind, Placebo-Controlled Study with a Standardized Hazelnut Extract," *Journal of Allergy and Clinical Immunology* 116 (2005): 1073–9.

8. S. H. Sicherer, "Clinical Implications of Cross-reactive Food Allergens." *Journal of Allergy and Clinical Immunology* 108 (2001): 881–8.

Chapter 11: Your Better Breathing Program

1. Andrew Weil, *Spontaneous Healing: How to Discover and Enhance Your Body's Natural Ability to Maintain and Heal Itself* (New York: Knopf, 1995).
2. Robert Fulford with Gene Stone, *Dr. Fulford's Touch of Life* (New York: Pocket Books, 1996).
3. Dean Ornish, *Dr. Dean Ornish's Program for Reversing Heart Disease: The Only System Scientifically Proven to Reverse Heart Disease without Drugs or Surgery* (New York: Random House, 1990).
4. Jon Kabat-Zinn, *Full Catastrophe Living: Using the Wisdom of your Body and Mind to Face Stress, Pain, and Illness* (New York: Delacorte, 1990).
5. Herbert Benson, *The Relaxation Response* (New York: Morrow, 1975).
6. John Sarno, *Healing Back Pain: The Mind-Body Connection* (New York: Warner Books, 1991).
7. Candace B. Pert, *Molecules of Emotion: Why You Feel the Way You Feel* (New York: Scribner, 1997).
8. Bill Moyers, *Healing and the Mind.* The Brain and the Immune System by David Felton p. 213. (New York: Doubleday, 1993).
9. M. Rosenkranz, W. Busse, T. Johnstone, et al., "Neural Circuitry Underlying the Interaction between Emotion and Asthma Symptom Exacerbation," *Proceedings of the National Academy of Sciences* 102 (2005): 13319–24.
10. R. C. de Charms, F. Maedo, G. H. Glover, et al., " Control Over Brain Activation and Pain Learned by Using Real Time Functional MRI." PNAS 102, no. 51 (December 20, 2005): 1862–3.
11. Debra Yemenijian, "The Story on Stress: Researchers Offer Insights About Asthma's Connection to Anxiety," *Advance* 14 (2005): 36.
12. Ibid.

13. Lyle H. Miller, Atma Dell Smith, Larry Rothstein, *The Stress Solution* (New York: Pocket Books. 1993).

14. Kobasa S. C., Maddi Sr. and Puccetti M. C.,: "Personality and Exercise as Buffers in the Stress Illness Relationship," *Journal of Behavioral Medicine* 5 (1982): 391–404.

15. Jon Kabat-Zinn, *Wherever You Go, There You Are.* (New York: Hyperion. 1994).

16. L. F. Berkman and S. L. Syme, "Social Networks, Host Resistance and Mortality: A Nine-Year Follow-up Study of Almeda County Residents," *American Journal of Epidemiology* 109 (1979): 186–204.

17. Thich Nhat Hanh, *Peace Is Every Step: The Path of Mindfulness in Everyday Life* (New York: Bantam Books, 1992).

18. S. C. Jain, L. Rai, A. Valedcha, et al., "Effect of Yoga Training on Exercise Tolerance in Adolescents with Childhood Asthma." *Journal of Asthma* 28, no. 6 (1991): 437–42.

19. Esther Myers, *Yoga and You: Energizing and Relaxing Yoga for New and Experienced Students* (Boston: Shambhala, 1997).

Index

winter allergy, 24
World Health Organization
(WHO), 73

X
Xolair, 48

Y
yoga, 156, 172–80
Yoga and You, 172

Z
Zyrtec-D, 43